Medicine
for the
Backcountry

by Buck Tilton and
Frank Hubbell

Enjoy the outdoors with many adventures

Frank Hubbell

Illustrations by
Marc Bohne

ICS BOOKS, INC.
Merrillville, Indiana

Medicine in the Backcountry
Copyright © 1990 by Buck Tilton and Frank Hubbell

Printed in U.S.A.

Published by:
ICS Books, Inc.
One Tower Plaza
107 E. 89th Avenue
Merrillville, IN 46410

Library of Congress Cataloging-in-Publication Data

Tilton, Buck.
    Medicine for the backcountry / by Buck Tilton and Frank Hubbell ; illustrations by Marc Bohne.
        p.   cm.
      ISBN 0-934802-61-0   : $9.95
      1. Mountaineering--Accidents and injuries. 2. First aid in illness and injury.   I. Hubbell, Frank   II. Title
    RC1220.M6T55   1990
    616.02'52--dc20   89-71636
                                                                       CIP

TABLE OF CONTENTS

SECTION IV. WILDLIFE HAZARDS

SECTION V. MEDICAL EMERGENCIES

SECTION VI. COMMON BACKCOUNTRY MEDICAL PROBLEMS

PREFACE

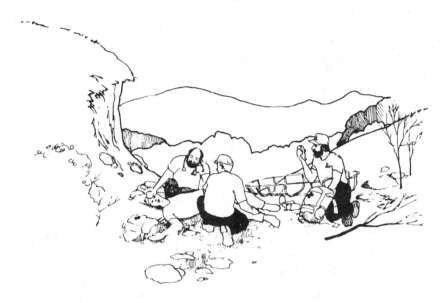

Rugged miles and tired muscles, the cutting edge of an icy wind, loose footing through a black night, all are a part of providing backcountry emergency care. Staying warm is a matter of the clothes you wear, the food you eat, the water you carry on your back. There are never too many to bear the litter, but always more than enough opinions about the best way to go. Your creativity and determination are directly proportional to your success. When the vitals are stable, the splints secure, your adrenalin rush ebbs, but the work has just begun.

We want to do it because we love the wild places, and we feel compassion for the wonderful and crazy people who go there. We want to preserve the lives of both. The way of the unrestrained river becomes our way, the endless movement, the steady flow, the path of least resistance.

From this book you may acquire knowledge that will help you ease pain and save lives, but it is merely information. Everything presented here should be tempered with the wisdom that comes from experience. Your greatest skill is your ability to reason and judge, your best piece of equipment is your brain. To come from your training with a pocketfull of pat answers is to miss the point. No two backcountry situations are ever the same. Here is a written foundation to build on. Finding the best way to do something is not as important as finding a method that works.

More important than your selection of a text is your choice of instructors. A team rarely exceeds the strength of its leader, or a course the ability of its teacher. Look for someone who can translate windsong and the moan of an aching back into understandable words and experiences.

Study first to know yourself, second to accept yourself, and third to discipline yourself toward a higher level of performance. Be silent and listen. Grow aware. When you have learned to change what you know into perfect patient care in the wilderness, your journey has begun.

CHAPTER 1
PRIMARY ASSESSMENT

Introduction

Dancing across the high mountain meadow in a glistening swirl of clarity, the South Fork of the Little Wind River blocked the hikers from their chosen campsite. They could see it lying in the shade of tall pines, a flat spot begging for a couple of tents. Dropping their backpacks, four of them began to patiently remove their socks and replace their boots, preparing to wade. The fifth sized up the spacing of rocks, judging the feasibility of a hopping dash to the other side.

Making his decision, the impatient dasher tightened his hipbelt and started across. The last rock before dry land was wet from periodic surges of the river. When the backpacker's foot fell there, it found no purchase. Up went his feet and down went his lower back, thumping heavily against the rock, the pack absorbing some of the blow. He crawled the remaining few feet to shore, and collapsed on his side. When his friends waded hurriedly to his assistance, the damaged hiker was unable to rise, complaining of severe lower back pain.

It was fourteen miles to the nearest road, which was dirt and seldom used. It was late September, the water was very cold, and the ground wasn't much better. Darkness was on the verge of settling down. It was time for an application of Backcountry Medicine.

This situation calls for much more than First Aid. First Aid is a part of it, but its intention is, and always has been, stabilization of the injured person until they can be transferred to a medical facility for definitive care. Even highly-skilled prehospital personnel are trained to respond in the context of short-term care of the injured and sick.

The wilderness requires long-term care in medicine, just as it insists on a higher level of self-sufficiency in all areas of living beyond the amenities of civilization. In a remote geographical environment, the time/distance relationship of the incident and a medical center is one of three ingredients that add to First Aid. The second is the severity of the environment: cold, wet, wind, heat, darkness, rough terrain, shortages of potable water, and more. And finally, the lack of specialized equipment often demands creative improvisation on the part of the rescuer.

Survey the Scene

Doubled up in pain, unable to move, the hasty backpacker lay deep in the Wind River Mountains, obviously hurt. But there was no immediate danger . . . or was there? What should you be thinking about as you approach this person? What is your first concern for your injured friend?

If your answer was Airway, Breathing, or Circulation (the ABC's), you have made a mistake, perhaps a serious one! Your first thoughts at any rescue scene should be toward your own safety, and the safety of others with you.

Maxim: Never Create a Second Victim

The worst thing you can do at any scene is create a second victim. A quick check for immediate hazards needs to be made. When an accident occurs, whether someone is injured or not, the result is invariably a degree of confusion. Disorganization promotes the chance of further injury, and delays the start of adequate patient care.

In the Winds, those who hurried to the rescue wore heavy packs and walked on slippery rocks. September darkness brought a plunge in temperature. Everyone was damp from a sweaty hike. The victim was drenched in icy river water, and had already begun to tremble.

It is difficult to find a well-managed scene without a manager. Someone needs to take charge! If a leader has not been pre-arranged, the time it requires to choose one may be the most valuable moments in the rescue. The leader needs to maintain a high level of objectivity. Staying objective will allow the leader to check the accident area for acute or subtle dangers, which includes checking the approach to the victim for safety. Leadership involves assigning appropriate tasks to everyone, gathering information to make a plan of action, and observing to insure nothing is left undone.

Take a deep calming breath. Take charge of yourself first. If you are alone, order the tasks that must be done, and get to work. Don't just stand there.

We are accustomed to thinking of getting the maximum good out of a minimum of equipment. We learn to look at everything as a potential asset: packframes, ensolite pads, bandannas, tent poles. All of these items share the characteristic of inanimateness. It takes a person to make them perform a needed function. People are the most valuable resource. They can think, plan, put up a tent, make hot tea, build a splint, carry a litter. When a second victim is created, the party not only has twice as many problems to deal with, but also one less of its most valuable resources. The situation is more than twice as difficult!

Train yourself to check first for a safe scene. Pause as you approach the victim, look to the leader for organization, ask "Is this safe?" It usually is, but the one time it isn't, all the difference in success or failure can be made if you notice the danger.

Primary Survey

Airway and Breathing

Breathing is a fantastic process. Contraction of the diaphragm and intercostal muscles causes the size of the space inside the chest to increase. To fill the space, air rushes in through the nose or mouth, past the throat, down the trachea (windpipe) to the bronchi, where it goes either right or left, through bonchioles of ever-diminishing size to the alveoli. In the alveoli, oxygen passes easily through a semi-permeable membrane and into the blood. Carbon dioxide leaves the blood, collecting in the alveoli. When the muscles relax, the chest cavity decreases in size, and the air is pushed out, expelling the carbon dioxide.

Everything works fine as long as the pathway of the air is not obstructed. If the scene is safe, your next concern is your patient's airway.

A simple question, "Are you OK?", often elicits a response such as "No, you idiot, didn't you see me fall?", which may or may not be an appropriate answer, but at least we are assured your patient can breathe. If they do not respond, you must get your ear down near the opening of their airway, and look, listen, and feel for air exchange.

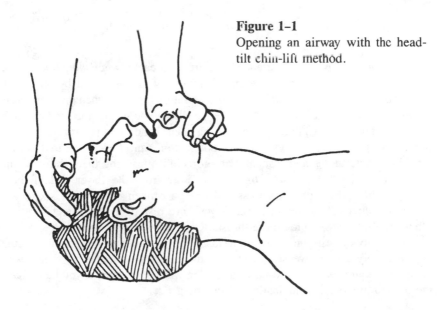

Figure 1–1
Opening an airway with the head-tilt chin-lift method.

The most common obstruction of the airway is the tongue. Deep unconsciousness can cause it, and the epiglottis, to fall back across the throat. An easy method for opening the airway is pushing down on the forehead while lifting the chin. Open the mouth of your patient and listen again for air movement. If there is a suspicion of neck injury, the airway can be opened with a lift of the jaw without movement of the neck.

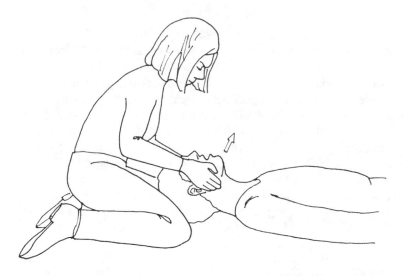

Figure 1–2
Opening an airway with the jaw thrust method.

On a good day, your patient will start to breathe when you open their airway. If they don't, it means either their airway is obstructed by an object other than their tongue, or they are in respiratory arrest. Pinching their nose closed, and sealing your mouth over theirs, allows you to breathe air into their lungs. If it won't go in, try repositioning their head, and attempt a second breath. No go? A foreign body airway obstruction can often be cleared out by straddling their thighs and manually and forcefully thrusting their abdomen up toward their chest. Keep your hands low, away from the lower end of their sternum where the xiphoid process waits to be broken off. Thrust six to ten times, and check their mouth to see if you have dislodged the object. Try another breath. Try six to ten more thrusts. Continue until it works.

A victim of respiratory arrest needs to have someone breathe for them, approximately every five seconds, until they start to breathe on their own. Mouth-to-mouth, or mouth-to-nose, breathing will work better if you have taken the time to practice in anticipation of an emergency.

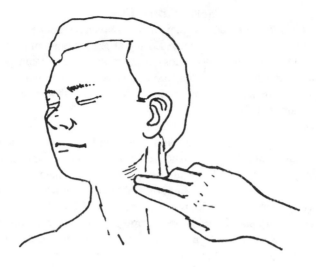

Figure 1–3
Checking the pulse at the carotid artery.

Circulation

The heart beats. The bloods goes round and round, leaving the heart through arteries, passing through capillaries, and returning through veins. Arteries carry de-oxygenated blood to the lungs, where it washes over the alveoli, discarding CO_2 and picking up fresh O_2. Arteries carry oxygenated blood to all of the body's seventy-five trillion or so cells. Every cell needs the oxygen to survive.

When your heart stops beating, you are clinically dead. In approximately four to six minutes, without oxygen, brain cells, the ones most easily effected by an O_2 shortage, begin to die. It doesn't take long for a significant number of brain cells to die, leaving you biologically dead.

During the few minutes between clinical and biological death, it is sometimes possible to interrupt the dying process and resuscitate the victim. It is, therefore, very important to assess the circulation of your patient as soon as possible. You can do that quickly by pressing several of your fingers lightly into the hollow below the angle of your patient's jaw. There you should feel the carotid pulse.

If you can not find the pulse, it is time to begin the process of chest compressions and mouth-to-mouth ventilations known as cardiopulmonary resuscitation (CPR). If you do not know how to perform CPR, you will very likely be wishing you had taken the time to learn.

Severe Bleeding

Once you reach your adult size, you probably have between five and six liters of blood circulating in your body. Losing about ten percent of it will cause you to feel weak and lightheaded. Loss of another ten to fifteen percent will result in inadequate perfusion of your tissues (see SHOCK) leaving you incapacitated until you can manufacture more blood. As blood loss approaches the fifty percent mark, the likelihood of death grows greater and greater.

It is important to check patients quickly for severe loss of blood. A visual scan is often enough. But sometimes blood loss can be hidden in bulky clothing and water-resistant shells. Check inside clothing if there is any possibility of severe bleeding. Heavy blood loss can also disappear into the environment upon which your patient is lying. Look underneath them in snow, sand, rocks, and any ground cover that may be hiding large amounts of blood.

Severe blood loss should be stopped immediately with pressure from your hand directly on the wound. Do not waste time looking for something to place over the wound first. Get in there and apply pressure. Direct pressure can be augmented by elevating the wound above the patient's heart.

Once pressure has been applied, it should be maintained until clotting is well established. If someone can get a bulky sterile dressing it can be tied firmly in place to maintain pressure. This pressure dressing should be monitored to make sure adequate circulation is getting past the pressure. You don't want it to become a tourniquet.

In some cases it isn't feasible to apply direct pressure. Perhaps the area is too large to compress, or the pressure causes your patient too much pain. Bleeding can be discouraged by putting pressure on pressure points. These are places where arteries are close enough to the surface to squash them against bone and reduce the flow of blood. The handiest two are 1) the brachial pressure point, anywhere inside the upper arm, and 2) the femoral, which lies along an imaginary line between the iliac crest (the high point of the pelvis) and the center of the groin.

Tourniquets cut off all blood flow and are used as last resorts. Tie it off and write it off. What you are writing off is the living tissue beyond the tourniquet. Flat material should be used (nylon webbing, for example) to prevent tearing of the skin. Any stick can be used to cinch the material down until blood flow stops.

The Cervical Spine

Fractures and dislocations of the seven bones that make up the neck, the cervical spine, can be repaired. Damage to the spinal cord running through them can not. The result of spinal cord damage in the cervical region is usually quadriplegia or death. For that reason we take the primary precaution of keeping the head and neck as still as possible if there is any suspicion of a cervical spine injury.

Our level of suspicion should be very high if the patient is unconscious or injured as a result of an accident which throws the neck forcefully out of alignment (falls from a height, sudden high-speed stops, blows to the head). They may or may not complain of neck pain. Sometimes spinal injuries ruin the life of a victim hours after the accident through subsequent swelling and movement.

Do not let fear of spinal injury blind you to more immediate threats to life. If the scene is not safe, the patient may need to be carefully moved (see SPINAL CORD INJURY MANAGEMENT). If the airway is not open, grasp the sides of your patient's head firmly, and pull with steady, gentle traction and attempt to align the head and neck with the rest of the body. Gentle traction should be maintained until mechanical stabilization can be improvised (see SPINAL CORD INJURY MANAGEMENT).

Maxim: When in Doubt, Treat the Worst Possible Injury.

The goal of the primary assessment is a patient who is initially safe from immediate threats to life. After being stabilized and moved to the warm security of a tent and sleeping bag, our Wind River victim lay for four uncomfortable days until a helicopter evacuation was accomplished. His recovery was eventually complete.

The Barehanded Principles:
Primary Assessment

1. *Check the scene for safety.*
2. *If in doubt about the cervical spine, manually stabilize it.*
3. *Ensure an airway and breathing.*
4. *Ensure the heart is circulating blood.*
5. *Stop any severe bleeding.*

CHAPTER 2
SECONDARY ASSESSMENT

Introduction

It was late afternoon, and northern New Hampshire grew chilly. With numbing hands, the climber on Cannon Mountain lost control and took a leader fall of approximately sixty feet, penduluming backfirst into the granite wall. Conscious, but unable to continue up or down, he was skillfully lowered to the ground by his partner, who ran for help.

When we arrived with a carrying team, he complained of head and chest pain, and had forgotten the specifics of what happened. Stabilized in the litter, we started out slowly, picking our way over the darkening pile of rubble at the foot of the route.

"How's the ride?" Frank asked our patient for the tenth time. But now he failed to get the irritated answer he expected. We stopped for a quick reassessment. The injured climber responded sluggishly to a painful stimulus. His respirations were deeper than the last check, and more labored. There was a significant increase in his blood pressure. Frank voiced all our concerns: "We're losing him."

Picking up the pace, stumbling in the bobbing light of headlamps, we hurried as best we could, reaching the trailhead in less time than we imagined possible. An exhausted team watched the ambulance pull briskly away.

The hospital at Littleton found nine ribs fractured near the spine and, more importantly, a swollen brain. Our notice of his deteriorating condition, and the following rush to the road, probably, said the attending physician, made the difference between death and the climber's fortunate recovery.

The Physical Exam

When the immediate threats to life have been controlled, our assessment needs to extend systematically over the entire patient, evaluating the extent of the known injuries, and looking for unsuspected damage hidden by the pain and the obvious. The situation will determine the sequence and thoroughness of this examination. But all patients deserve a complete, hands-on, head-to-toe check. (In a small child, you may wish to go toe-to-head, gaining their confidence before attacking their vulnerable head and chest.)

General guidelines for the patient exam include:
1. Gentle but firm palpation (feeling) of all relevant body parts, looking for obvious damage, pain responses, swelling, deformities, and abnormalities.
2. Moving the patient as little as possible, and not aggravating known injuries.
3. When necessary, cutting away clothing to visualize suspected injuries.
4. Communicating with the patient through the entire process, even if they appear unconscious. They are the questions, and they are the answers!

Specifically move from head to toe, Looking, Asking, and Feeling (LAF) for the signs and symptoms of problems. It is a kind way to LAF at them.

HEAD: Looking for damage, discoloration, and blood or fluid draining from ears, nose, and mouth. Asking about loss of consciousness, pain, or any abnormal sensations. Feeling for lumps or other deformities.

NECK: Looking for obvious damage, or deviance in the trachea. Asking about pain and discomfort. Feeling along the cervical spine for a pain response.

CHEST: Compress the ribs from both sides, as if squeezing a bird cage, keeping your hands wide to prevent the possibility of too much direct pressure on fractures. Look for damage or deformities. Ask about pain. Feel for unstability.

ABDOMEN: With hands spread wide, press gently on the abdomen. Look for damage. Ask about pain and discomfort. Feel for rigidity, distention, or muscle spasms.

BACK: Slide your hands under the patient, palpating as much of the spine as possible.

PELVIS: Cup the iliac crests with your hands, pressing gently down, and pulling toward the midline of the body. Ask about pain. Feel for instability.

LEGS: With your hands surrounding each leg, one at a time, run from the groin down to the toes, squeezing as you go. Note especially if there is a lack of circulation, sensation, or motion in the toes.

SHOULDERS AND ARMS: One at a time, with hands wide, squeeze each shoulder, and run down the arms to the fingers. Check for circulation, sensation, and motion in the fingers.

A conscious or dictated note of all possible injuries should be kept. Don't let known injuries keep you from a thorough examination. Soon you will be treating all suspected damage.

The Vital Signs

An accurate measurement of a body's vital functions do not tell you what is wrong with your patient. But they do relate how well your patient is doing. The second set of vital signs is more important than the first set. And the third more important that the second. Circumstances will dictate how often the signs are taken, but the change over time is the key to using vital signs in long-term patient care. A constant monitoring of your patient should be maintained until they are "out of the woods."

LEVEL OF CONSCIOUSNESS: A normal level of consciousness allows your patient to answer intelligently in a way that tells you he or she is oriented in person, place, and time. They should know who they are, where they are, and generally what time it is. The LOC is the easiest sign to assess, and the first to change. It can be recorded easily using the AVPU scale, which assigns the patient a letter grade from alert to unresponsive.

ALERT: The patient seems normal, and answers intelligently questions about person, place, and time. They know essentially what happened to them.

VERBAL: The patient is not Alert, but they do respond in some way when spoken to.

PAIN: The patient does not react to verbal stimuli, but they do react to being pinched or rubbed in sensitive areas.

UNRESPONSIVE: The patient does not respond to stimuli.

PULSE: In the Primary Assessment you noticed a pulse at the carotid artery, assuring yourself your patient had blood being pumped to the brain. Now you are interested in the rate, rhythm, and quality of that pulse. Using the radial pulse, inside the wrist, where the thumb side of the hand joins the arm, is much more comfortable for the patient than pressing their neck. Press lightly with several fingertips.

RATE: The number of beats per minute. A range of 60–80 is normal in an adult. It will usually be higher in children, sometimes reaching a norm of 160 in an infant. Counting for one full minute is more accurate, but a count for 15 seconds and multiplying by four is acceptable and most often used. In the absence of a watch, take a pulse anyway. At least you can assess the rhythm and quality.

RHYTHM: There will be either a clock-like regularity, or a sporadic irregularity.

QUALITY: This refers to the force exerted by the heart on each beat. The force will be best judged by its relation to previous pulse checks. A Normal quality is strong, a Thready pulse is weak and an indication of inadequate circulation, and a Bounding pulse is abnormally forceful.

An absence of a radial pulse is cause for alarm. But delay panicking until you check the other arm. The cause might be an injury to the arm or shoulder.

RESPIRATIONS: A patient alerted to the fact that you're checking their respirations may voluntary alter their breathing pattern. Keep your assessment a secret.

RATE: An adult normally breathes 12–18 times per minute. Children and infants breath faster.

RHYTHM: Normally, we breath evenly and regularly, exhalations taking slightly longer than inhalations. Watch for shallowness or deepness, and irregularities in the pattern.

QUALITY: Normal breathing is quiet and effortless. Abnormal breathing might include labor, pain, noise (snores, squeaks, gurgles, gasps), and a flaring of the nostrils.

SKIN: It's on the outside, away from the body's core where vital life processes are centered, but the skin gives pertinent information on the general well-being of our patient.

COLOR: Pink is the normal color of skin, pink in the non-pigmented areas of the body—the lining of the eye, inside the mouth, fingernail beds. It may be difficult to detect subtle changes in darker complexions, but the overall color of the skin is also an indicator. The size of the blood vessels near the skin determine color. Vasodilation (widening vessels) produces a red, flushed color, and indicates problems such as fever or hyperthermia. Vasocontriction (narrowing vessels) produces pale or blotchy skin, and may indicate shock or hypothermia. A blue hue, called cyanosis, shows a lack of oxygen, and often indicates heart failure. Yellowish skin tells of liver failure.

TEMPERATURE: The temperature of the skin can be significantly lower than the body's core and still be perfectly healthy. It will indicate, though, whether the patient is vasodilating and growing warmer, or vasocontricting and getting cooler.

MOISTURE: Normal skin is relatively dry. Warmth and wetness from excessive sweating may be evident, but if the skin is cool and moist, it may indicate shock.

BLOOD PRESSURE: BP's are impossible to take without a device called a sphygmomanometer, and are more accurate if you have a stethoscope as well. It is mentioned briefly here because of its importance, along with a very crude field assessment technique.

Your beating heart creates pressure on the walls of your blood vessels. Without that pressure within the circulatory system, the oxygen-carbon dioxide transfer would not take place down on a cellular level. When the pressure drops too low for perfusion and adequate oxygenation to occur, tissues begin to die, and soon the organism follows. Blood pressure has two components: 1) the systolic pressure, measured when the heart is contracting, and 2) the diastolic measured when the heart is at rest. A general norm is written as 120/80, but the pressure varies greatly from individual to individual.

As the pressure drops, skin becomes more and more cyanotic. Pulses begin to disappear. You'll lose the pulse in your feet first, then your wrist, and, finally, your neck. If you found the radial pulse of your patient earlier, and now it's gone, they are losing pressure.

The Medical History

As you practice, you will gain pride in your ability to perform a patient exam and take a set of vital signs. But the tricky part of assessment, and probably 80% of your final verdict, will come from the information gathered as you interview your patient.

Approach with a calm, confident attitude, whether you feel it or not. An aura of calmness surrounding the scene will often do more for the sick and injured than all the splints and aspirin you can throw at them. Quietly say, "Hi, I read a book on Backcountry Medicine and I can help you." Don't scream, "What happened, what happened?"

If you haven't already, establish a relationship with your patient. It is more effective to say sincerely, "I know you must be afraid and in pain, but we'll make you as comfortable as possible," as opposed to panting, "You'll be OK, you'll be fine."

Create a positiveness about the situation. Say, "Are you more comfortable sitting up or lying down?" Don't say, "Which hurts more?"

Be enthusiastic without being a cheerleader. Be kind without being nauseating. Be honest without saying everything you're thinking. Beware of the tone of your voice. Beware of your patient's tendency to take the slightest offhand comment as truth. Discuss with them the possible plans of action. They have a right to their say in what happens.

A helpful mnemonic is AMPLE:

ALLERGIES: "Are you allergic to anything you know of?"

MEDICATIONS: "Taking anything currently?"

PAST HISTORY: "Is there anything possibly relevant I should know about your health?" Or, "Has anything like this happened before?"

LAST MEAL: "When did you eat or drink last?"

EVENTS: "What led up to this?" And finally, "Is there anything else I should know?"

The questions you ask should not lead the patient on. Don't ask, "Is it a sharp pain?" Ask instead, "Can you describe the pain for me?"

If they are in pain or discomfort, another mnemonic is PQRST. What, if anything, PROVOKES the pain? What is the QUALITY of the pain? Does it RADIATE? Describe the SEVERITY? And what TIME did the problem start?

If your patient is unconscious, you have to become even more of a Sherlock Holmes in your search for clues. Are they wearing Medical Alert tags on neck, wrists, ankles? Is there information in their pockets? What can you learn from witnesses? From anyone around who knows them? What evidence does the scene hold for you? Seek answers to the AEIOU TIPS: Is their unconsciousness the result of ALLERGIES, EPILEPSY, INFECTION, OVERDOSE, UNDER-DOSE, TRAUMA, INSULIN, PSYCHOLOGICAL disorder, STROKE.

The SOAP Note

When time allows, or if there are spare hands at the scene, all the information gathered during the assessment, and what was done for treatment, should be recorded on paper. You will never remember everything, vital signs slip away like autumn leaves in a high wind, and the patient deserves to have any physician who later takes over know the details of what happened and what was done. The note also becomes a legal record if a medicolegal question arises. Even if you're not sure what you're doing is absolutely correct, you want to record all your efforts in the patient's behalf. It shows you did your best.

The note can be divided into four sections for convenience of memory:

SUBJECTIVE: What happened to who (include age, address, and sex) where, and when? What is their chief complaint?

OBJECTIVE: What did the physical exam reveal? What are the vital signs, and when did you do the following checks? What is the relevant medical history?

ASSESSMENT: What are the possible problems?

PLAN: What are you going to do?

Eventually you'll add to the note your name, and the names of any other members of the aiding party, and witnesses.

The Barehanded Principles: Secondary Assessment

1. Create an aura of calmness and confidence.

2. Do a complete, head-to-toe physical examination.

3. *Check (and keep checking) the vital signs: level of consciousness, pulse, respirations, skin.*
4. *Take a medical history.*
5. *Write a SOAP note.*

CHAPTER 3
SHOCK

Introduction

Our camp was set on the Muddy Boo after a long day of simmering in Old Town Trippers. It was Florida, it was August, it was hot, and it was humid. The canoes were cleaned, and lashed to trees near the river. Dinner was over, and darkness settled over the camp like an electric blanket trained to kill.

Final instructions were given to the kids: "Don't leave your tents without your shoes. This is mean country, ready to take a bite out of you in many ways!" We were the last to zip up our doors against the descending horde of night marauders.

We called him Sugar Dog because he acted sweet but was ready to take a nip out of your backside if you turned. He left his tent deep in the night, without his shoes of course, when his brain lost an argument with his bladder over a question of urination. His half-muffled scream came from the least of our concerns. No snakes, spiders, scorpions. No 'gators or wild pigs or rabid skunks. No broken glass or rusty shards of old cans. The Dog had thumped his big toe against a partially buried log.

The initial response to being injured is the same for all humans. A message runs from the site of the injury, in this case the big toe, to the brain. It is not an "ouch" message. It is an "alert" message, informing the brain something bad is happening. The brain throws the body into an alert status, preparing to deal with the problem. The heart rate speeds up, and blood rushes out to the body faster. The respiratory rate increases, keeping the blood enriched with oxygen. The skin turns pale and clammy as the vessels near the edge of the body constrict to increase circulation to the vital inner organs. If you were watching Sugar Dog, your first indication something was wrong would be a change in his level of consciousness—he would appear anxious, a reflection of his brain's concern over the unknown extent of the injury.

With the vital processes secure, in seconds, the brain asks the toe: "What's going on down there?"

The toe says, "You stubbed me viciously. I'm probably broken!"

"That's it?" asks the brain. "Nothing life-threatening?"

"It seemed important at the time," says the toe, now embarrassed over the commotion.

"What a wimp," mumbles the brain, and relaxes the alert status. Sugar Dog looks relieved, his heart slows down, he takes a deep slow breath, his normal color returns. The toe, in one last act of defiance over the brain's control, starts to throb as the nerve passageways return to normal.

We found The Dog sitting on the ground, holding his toe, and cursing. It only took a moment to assess him as relatively uninjured, and to begin our own cursing over his flagrant disregard for the rules.

If we had found a cause for real concern, let's say a deep gash in an artery of his lower leg, we would have had to handle the problem and the possibility of a serious sequel to the problem—shock.

Normal Physiology

Your cardiovascular system (heart, vessels, and blood) is really two circulatory systems joined at the heart. The right side of the heart pumps blood to the lungs and back. The left side pushes oxygen-rich blood to all parts of the body and back. Both circuits work simultaneously. Cardiac output, the amount of blood pumped out by the heart every minute, is normally enough to meet the needs of all the cells of your body.

Blood leaves the heart through arteries, that branch and narrow to arterioles, that branch and narrow to capillaries. At the capillaries, the oxygen (and nutrients picked up from the digestive system) are diffused across cell walls, exchanged for carbon dioxide and the waste products of metabolism. The waste-carrying blood moves out the other end of the capillaries, into venules that come together to form veins. The veins return blood to the heart. Veins are more numerous than arteries, and can hold more of your blood. There is less pressure in the veins, and they have little one-way doors to keep the blood from backing up. All vessels can dilate or constrict to meet varying demands from the body.

Your body's systems are designed to support the lives of your cells. When cellular life cannot be maintained, death of the organism occurs. The constant bathing of cells with life-sustaining fluid under proper pressure is called *perfusion*.

Shock

Shock is an inadequate perfusion of the body's cells with oxygenated blood. It results when cardiac output is too low to keep the cells washed with enough blood under enough pressure to allow diffusion to take place. Shock can be caused by failure of one or more of the three parts of the cardiovascular system. 1) HYPOVOLEMIC SHOCK is a result of loss of fluid from the system. It can be produced by external or internal blood loss, plasma loss from burns, or dehydration from diarrhea, vomiting, and excessive sweating. 2) CAR-DIOGENIC SHOCK is a result of "pump failure" leading to a decrease in blood flow and a fall in blood pressure. 3) NEUROGENIC (Vasogenic) SHOCK results when the resistance of the muscular vessel walls relax and blood pools in the veins, returning to the heart at an inadequate level. This can come from damage or excitation to the central nervous system, bodywide infection, or a severe allergic reaction.

Shock is a progressive problem, passing through three stages on its way to causing death. 1) During the COMPENSATORY STAGE, the body compensates for the damage by increasing its activity level. 2) The PROGRESSIVE STAGE begins when the compensatory mechanisms fail, and the condition of the patient declines, often rapidly. 3) The IRREVERSIBLE STAGE is reached when inadequate perfusion results in the cells of vital organs starting to die, when even the most definitive measures may not save the patient.

Whatever the cause, shock victims share similar signs and symptoms, all deriving from inadequate perfusion. Their level of consciousness is one of ANXIETY and RESTLESSNESS, from inadequate perfusion of the brain, progressing to unconsciousness and coma. Their HEART RATE INCREASES, and often feels weak and thready. ABNORMAL RESPIRATIONS, usually quick and shallow, progress to labored. They SWEAT heavily, the skin feeling COOL AND CLAMMY, and progressively becoming cyanotic or ashen gray in color. They often complain of THIRST from dehydration, and NAUSEA from inadequate perfusion of the stomach. The progressive stage will lead to DULL EYES and a BLOOD PRESSURE DROP.

The severity of shock is relative to the extent of the injury, and whether or not the cause can be treated. For the patient to be treated successfully in the backcountry, early recognition and management are essential!

Maxim: Assume Shock in All Patients with Injury or Illness.

Treatment of Shock

The primary goal in the treatment of shock is the same as with any patient—secure and maintain an airway. If there is a cause that can be treated (as in direct pressure on severe bleeding), do it. Since your patient is suffering from an insufficiency of oxygen, it would be wonderful if you could give them supplemental oxygen, but that is most often not possible in the wilderness. It is very important to keep them calm and reassured! Have them lie down, if they aren't already, and elevate their feet about a foot if the elevation does not aggravate an injury. Elevation increases blood flow to the vital organs. (Cardiogenic shock is an exception to the lie-down-and-elevate principle. They usually feel better sitting up, reducing the strain on their heart.) Keep them warm. Anticipate the worst, and begin immediate plans for evacuation to a medical facility. Unless the evacuation is very long, do not give the patient anything to eat or drink. The possibility of vomiting is high and dangerous. Small amounts of food, and especially water, might necessarily be given over a long evacuation, if the patient is alert and able to accept a cup and drink from it.

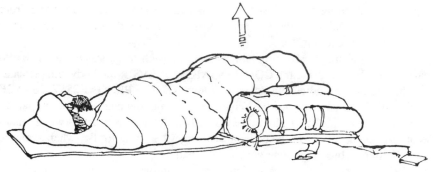

Figure 3–1
Shock treatment position.

The Barehanded Principles:
Shock

1. *Assume shock until proven otherwise.*
2. *Maintain an adequate airway.*
3. *Treat the cause if possible.*
4. *Keep the patient calm and reassured.*
5. *Keep the patient lying down with feet elevated unless shock is cardiogenic.*
6. *Keep the patient warm.*
7. *Do not give food and water unless absolutely necessary, and the patient is alert.*
8. *Monitor the patient closely for changes.*
9. *Plan an immediate evacuation.*

CHAPTER 4
SPINAL CORD
INJURY MANAGEMENT

Introduction

Murray and I are making our way down the steep slope of Denali Pass. Stretched below us on the snow are two victims, one stirring, the other motionless. Our intention was to summit on this unusually clear Alaskan day. We saw the two climbers ahead of us fall, tumbling six hundred feet, head-over-heels. One pack flew off. The glint of an ice axe arched through the air, still attached to the climber's wrist.

There is blood on the snow, leaking from where the axe cut a hole in the face of the unconscious victim. He is breathing rapidly with grunting moans on exhalation. Primary surveys reveal the other patient is likely to have suffered no serious injury, but the unconscious moaner reacts to pain in his head and neck. It is the kind of scenario you hate most: a possible cervical spine injury deep in the wilderness.

The human spine is a marvelously intricate structure of 33 bones (vertebrae) that give support yet flexibility to the body. By restricting motion to within definite bounds, the bones provide protection for the delicate spinal cord, the super-highway of nerves running down the center of the vertebrae.

The top seven bones of the spine work with the muscles of the neck to support the head. These cervical vertebrae are the smallest and most flexible in the spinal column, and, as you might expect, are the most susceptible to injury. Next, twelve thoracic vertebrae have ribs attached to them, helping to form the chest cavity that holds the heart and lungs. The lower back is composed of five lumbar vertebrae, the largest components of the spine. Since the last two thoracic vertebrae are attached to ribs that float freely in front (not being attached to the sternum), that region of the spine (T-10 to L-1) gives us more rotational freedom, and consequently is another high risk area for injury. Below the lumbar spine a lump of bones called the sacrum holds on to the pelvis. Finally the little coccyx reminds us, perhaps, that we once extended farther in that direction. The fused bones of the sacrum and coccyx gives us the total of 33. The spinal cord becomes loosely connected strings of nerves, like a horse's tail, in the lumbar region, and ends before the sacrum.

Types of Spinal Cord Injuries

1. The Uninterrupted Spinal Cord: There may be broken vertebrae, or there may not. There may be torn supporting ligaments in the spine. But the cord itself is not damaged. The patient needs to be carefully handled to insure the cord remains uninterrupted.

2. The Partial Spinal Cord Injury: There are probably fractures and definitely swelling that interrupts the blood supply to the cord. The result is loss of some motor function in the arms and/or legs, some loss of feeling, and some weakness. A partial injury can progress to a full one.

3. The Full Spinal Cord Injury: There is a severe interruption of spinal cord function.

Assessing the Injury

Once the scene is safe, and the primary assessment is completed, include a neurologic checkup in your secondary. Ask the patient to wiggle their toes, and have them press against your hand with their feet as against the accelerator of a car, and then the opposite motion, lifting their feet against pressure from your hand. Ask them to wiggle their fingers, and squeeze a finger of your hand. Spinal cord injury can affect their ability to do one or more of these things. A neck injury may produce difficulty breathing and the signs and symptoms of shock.

In the patient exam, check carefully for pain and tenderness in the neck.

Assessing a patient thoroughly includes gathering information about the forces, movement, and materials involved in the traumatic event. These insights become even more significant when evaluating a possible spinal injury. Some victims with seriously injured spines will get up and walk, complaining of no pain or loss of movement until permanent paralysis sets in. Your job as a rescuer is to recognize the chance of an injury, and treat the patient accordingly.

Any mechanism forcing the spine out of its normal range of motion or overloading it beyond its ability to bear weight can cause a serious injury. Of specific concern are violent flexion motions (especially chin to chest), violent rotations, and loads that compress the spine. Accidents commonly providing this type of violence in the backcountry are falls from a height and diving injuries. Even when the faller lands on their feet, the spine can compress excessively, and certainly if they land in a sitting position. A diver who hits a submerged object, or even one who hits the water wrong, can overload and over-flex their spine. Excessive flexion can occur when a skier hits a tree at high speed. A less common but devastating spinal injury called a distraction (the opposite of compression) is possible when a climber falls and momentarily dangles from a rope or rack. And, of course, a combination of factors may be at work in the accident.

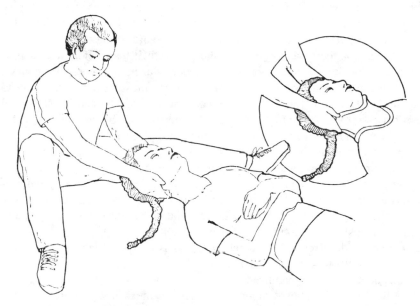

Figure 4–1
Manual stabilization of a possible neck injury.
(Inset: cervical collar.)

Managing the Spinal Injury

The goal is to prevent any further injury, and to do it the neck and spinal cord need to be immobilized and stabilized. Your immediate care should include telling your patient to lie still! An extra set of hands immobilizing the patient's head is very useful. Whether the patient is lying, sitting, or standing, someone should move to their rear and take gentle but firm control of their neck by holding on to the head.

But what if the scene isn't safe? What if an avalanche is pouring down the mountainside? What if they're lying half in an icy cold stream? Getting the patient to a safe place must take precedence over injury to their spine, but not at the exclusion of the spine. The answer is Body Elevation and Movement (BEAM). Get as many hands on the patient as possible, with firm ones on the head. At the command of the head immobilizer, lift the patient *as a unit*. BEAM them to a safe place without moving the spine from the position you found it in.

If the patient lies unconscious, you must first assume a neck injury until it is proven otherwise. If the neck lies at an odd angle, it should be straightened before treatment is continued. This can be accomplished safely with gentle traction-in-line, by pulling steadily and slowly on the head along the line in which you find the neck. Then move the neck to the neutral position, the spine in a line. To provide this movement with the utmost safety for your patient, it is best to see it done by someone who knows how before trying it yourself.

A patient on their side can be log-rolled on to their back before treatment is continued. Traction should be applied to the neck during movement. Of course, a log-roll can move a patient to their side if a pad must be put under them to keep the cold ground from eating their body heat. With the pad in place, roll them back on to it. (If your group is small, the pad can be used as a sled for moving the patient to a safer or more comfortable place.)

With the spine in the neutral position, the next step is to stabilize the cervical spine in place. Ambulances carry a cervical collar, a device that wraps around the neck to prevent excessive movement, especially the deadly chin-to-chest flexion. In the backcountry, extra clothing can be wrapped carefully around the patient's neck. Better yet, cut the end off an ensolite sleeping pad to fit the patient's neck, and tie or tape it in place.

Do not be deceived into thinking the collar is adequate stabilization. Manual, hands-on attention to the neck must still be maintained until the whole body of the patient can be immobilized on a rigid support. This rigid support takes the form of a full backboard in an ambulance. In the wilds, you are probably looking at a long wait for someone to go for help. Your patient needs to be made Free Of Any Movement (FOAM) in an unflexible litter. FOAMing is very difficult to accomplish with an improvised litter. It has been done by lashing external pack frames together with great attention to detail, and lashing dry limbs from the forest floor together with even greater attention to detail. (Green limbs flex too much!) In winter, skis may possibly be used to construct a rigid sled for the transportation of a spinal injury.

Once a litter is available, it is critical to FOAM the body of the patient in place (lots of padding and many straps) before tying down the head. A sudden movement of the patient with the head tied down and the body not can cause all you've been trying so hard to prevent. The body straps should include the shoulders. They work best if the straps crisscross the patient's chest putting less strain on the diaphragm while holding the torso securely down. The head should be padded and tied or taped to the litter.

As with any patient, but certainly with this one, you need to keep calm communication going with this helpless person you're lashing to a rack of torture. Look for places the rope, or tubular webbing, or whatever you're using, may be biting into the patient, and pad there. Pad in places the rigid support may produce painful pressure, like behind the knees.

Proceed with great care. Permanent spinal injuries are often the result of improper handling on the scene.

The Barehanded Principles:
Spinal Cord Injury Management

1. *Secure the Scene, by BEAMing the patient if necessary.*
2. *Secure the Airway, by Traction-in-Line movement of the cervical spine if necessary.*
3. *Improvise a Cervical Collar.*
4. *Keep hands-on maintenance to prevent uncontrolled movement of the spine.*
5. *Go for (or in desperation, Improvise) a rigid litter.*
6. *FOAM the patient on the litter for careful evacuation.*

CHAPTER 5
SOFT TISSUE INJURIES

Introduction

Even in July the Wind River Mountains are a chilly place. It was a classic, cold Rocky Mountain morning that found David and Bobby standing at the base of the Southwest Ridge of Nylon Peak, on the Continental Divide. By the time David began to inch his way up the initial pitch, his hands were truly numb. At some point along the rope length, cold flesh overgripped sharp granite. As the angle eased, David shook his hands for warmth and felt his own blood slap against his cheek. This was the first he knew of the damage to his fingers. He arrived at the belay with a left hand covered in blood, displaying at least six magnificent flaps of avulsed skin, two each on the pinky, ring, and middle fingers.

Once off the climb, Bobby trimmed the ragged, filthy tissue, leaving six open wounds. Lots of soap and water left him satisfied, and David grimacing. David spent ten days on a daily routine of wash/air-out/cover/uncover/re-wash/ air-out. He hiked with the hand bandaged and inside a nylon overmitt. By the end of the trip he had some dry scabs, some new pink skin, and was well on his way to being able to make a fist again.

Our skin does a lot of great things for us. It is essential in regulating the inner temperature of our bodies, which must be carefully controlled for us to stay alive. It oils itself to maintain flexibility, so we don't dry up and split open. It provides a sensory avenue, allowing us to intimately contact the world around us. But we are concerned here with the skin as a waterproof layer, keeping inside fluid in and outside fluid out, and the skin as protection against a wide world of bacteria waiting vigilantly to invade us.

You'd think Mother Nature, in all her infinite wisdom, would have made us tougher on the outside where the wear and tear takes place. Not so! We are forever abusing our skin with bashes, scrapes, nicks, slices, and impalements, opening our defenses to blood loss and any germ who happens to be crawling past. Knowing how to manage injuries to skin, and the underlying layers of fat and muscle, is a significant part of providing adequate backcountry care.

Wound Management

Any disruption in the vasculature of our bodies results in a bleeding wound. The immediate severity of the injury depends on the number of vessels we disrupt, and whether they are spurting arteries, flowing veins, or oozing capillaries. Sometimes the damage is internal (a bruise, a sprain, a broken bone) and the bleeding is characterized by swelling and discoloration. Sometimes the damage is external and characterized by blood running out and making a mess.

Our natural response to being opened in unnatural places is a remarkable and involuntary attempt to return to a balanced internal state. There is a prompt constriction of the tissue around the wound, compressing the small vessels and slowing blood loss. For ten minutes or so the vasculature of our entire body will constrict reducing blood loss even more. Attracted to the site of the injury, the platelets in our blood form plugs in the torn vessels. A process called coagulation builds a clot of elastic protein filaments restoring the integrity of the vasculature until full healing occurs. It is a wonderful thing that even small furry mammals can do.

You, as a rescuer, want to have three goals in handling a wound: 1) Stop the Bleeding, 2) Prevent Infection, and 3) Promote Healing.

99.99% of all bleeding can be stopped with direct pressure and elevation. Apply the pressure with your hand directly on the site of the injury, and elevate the wound above the patient's heart. Sometimes it is necessary to remove or cut away clothing to get a good look at the injured area. It is best to get a sterile dressing from your first aid kit to place on the wound before applying pressure, but, if the bleeding is serious, jump in right away with your dirty, greasy, grimy hand and stop the blood loss. If the bleeding is slow, it is perfectly OK to let it go for a few minutes, which actually cleans out the wound a bit. Keep the patient in a restful position, and avoid any unnecessary movement for at least the time it takes for the natural plug to form.

Direct pressure and elevation are contraindicated in places where the injury could be made worse by those actions. These places include:
1) a patient's neck where you might cut off their air supply. Neck bleeds can usually be stopped by pinching carefully around the opening with your fingers.
2) a patient's skull where you might push cracked bone into their brain. Open head wounds tend to bleed ferociously because the vessels in the scalp don't spasm and seal themselves off as they do in thinner skinned areas of the body. If there is a suspicion of skull fracture, place bulky sterile dressings over the wound and apply light pressure. When that doesn't work, pull the

edges of the wound together and tape it closed. Bandages designed for holding wound edges together work best, but any tape might do.

The prevention of infection almost equates with proper wound cleaning. A
healthy cleaning also speeds healing and reduces scarring. The basic techniques
include scrubbing, irrigation, and debridement.

Start by carefully washing your own hands. Avoid breathing into, coughing
around, or drooling all over an open wound. Scrubbing is to clean thoroughly
around, and sometimes inside, the wound. It is preferable to use an antiseptic
preparation created for wound cleaning (povidone-iodine, benzalkonium chloride, hexachlorophene), but soap and clean water, or just clean water, can be
used if nothing better is available. Scrub with a sterile gauze pad away from the
open injury. Scrubbing can be used directly on the surface of the wound if
foreign material is embedded there. Finally, rinse out anything that falls into the
wound, including the antiseptic preparation created for wound cleaning. Anything left in the wound retards healing.

The purpose of irrigation is to remove contaminants from the wound surface. A high pressure stream of an acceptable solution is directed into the opening. Optimally, you would use a syringe and needle, or an irrigation syringe,
with sterile saline solution. You can use any sort of clean plastic bag with a
pinhole punched in it, and water with a disinfectant added (like iodine). Or just
shoot some clean water into the wound if that's all you have.

Technically, debridement is the removal of visualized foreign particles and
dead tissue. Any foreign matter that does not come out with irrigation can be
picked out with discrimination and tweezers you have sterilized in boiling water.
Or scrub as explained earlier. A guideline for dead tissue removal is: Trimming
dead tissue causes no pain.

Follow scrubbing, irrigation, and debridement with a final flush using an
appropriate solution, and you are ready to promote healing. If you have properly
cleaned the wound, an antiseptic ointment may actually gum up the works and
retard healing. Let small wounds dry in the sunshine and clean air before dressing them. Larger wounds, the ones on their way to a doctor, will probably be
best dressed moist to prevent excessive drying out that could interfere with
definitive treatment. If the wound gapes open, and you're going to be many
hours getting out of the woods, pull the edges of the injury as neatly together as
possible, and tape it closed.

Specific Wounds

Bruises. Or contusions, as the erudite like to call them, are pockets of blood
collecting in soft tissue after a blow or a tearing motion (as in twisting a joint too
far). Torn blood vessels produce the color, and the pain and swelling is relative
to the severity of the injury. Bruises are an example of a closed wound, one not
open to the outside world.

They are usually minor, but a big bruise can be treated with an application of RICE (Rest, Ice, Compression, Elevation). After about 48 hours, heat can be applied to stimulate healthy circulation.

Abrasions. A piece of skin has been rubbed or scraped away, leaving a weeping raw spot that hurts a lot. The pain can be very bothersome because nerve endings (those receptors responsible for the ouch of an injury) are near the surface and not buried in fat or muscle. This type of wound is often dirty.

Convince the patient of the efficacy of letting you scrub the area clean. Once the wound has dried a dressing is not necessary except to protect the spot from further bumps and scrapes. If you do dress it, be sure that blood and other body fluids have stopped leaking out or else the dressing will become one with the body. Then you'll have to soak it off later.

Lacerations. The skin has been opened in either a neat or ragged line. After the bleeding has stopped, and the wound is clean, it might sag open. You will have less bother with it (and it'll heal faster) if you pull it closed with a tape bandage designed for that purpose. If you pull a laceration closed, you must watch it closely for signs of infection. It is easy to trap germs in a closed wound outside a sterile hospital environment. They like it in there. They want to be kept moist and warm where they grow best. If you have the material, it would be wise to re-wash the wound every day, and put on a fresh dressing.

If the wound gapes open horribly, it is usually best to bandage it open, leaving an antiseptic soaked piece of gauze in the wound to keep the drainage process going while you evacuate the patient.

Consider seeing a doctor for all gaping wounds, large or small, to be checked for underlying damage, and infection, and for stitches to reduce scarring.

Avulsions. Where something has sliced in at an angle, leaving a piece of flesh that lifts away from the rest of the body. If possible, replace the flap before applying direct pressure. After cleaning, this little "trapdoor" should be bandaged back in as close to its original position as possible. The wound will be less sensitive, and the avulsed piece might grow back into place. If the avulsed part is hopelessly de-circulated, it will die. If it is small and ratty, sometimes trimming off the ragged ends is OK before bandaging. Otherwise, wait to see if the piece survives before hacking away at it.

Amputations. Sometimes the avulsed part is totally separated from the body at the time of the injury. Even small parts, like the tip of a finger, can often be replaced successfully in the emergency room, often several hours after the accident. The salvage process requires the proper handling of the amputated part. It needs to be kept moist and cold, but not wet and frozen. For the backcountry, the technique most likely to work would be wrapping the part in slightly moist sterile gauze, putting the gauze in a sealable plastic bag, and putting the bag in

ice water. Any combination of the above is better than letting it dry out un-
wrapped or swell up from being too wet. Even if you have no hope for the
amputated piece of person, packing it out is probably an act of kindness.

Punctures. Human skin, being elastic, immediately closes around whatever
stuck into it, effectively cleaning off a load of germs and dirt when the puncturing object pulls out. If you get there soon enough, irritating a small puncture
wound, encouraging it to bleed, is OK. Scrub the area, and squirt an iodine
solution as deeply into the hole as possible, attempting to attack the embedded
bacteria. Without iodine, irrigate the wound with water, at least a liter of it. Do
not close the wound with tape or a tight bandage, or smear an ointment over it.
The wound needs to drain. A large puncture wound can have a piece of sterile
gauze left in it for a couple of days to hold it open in order to encourage
draining.

Puncture wounds can be insidious, a minor wound on the surface with
major damage hidden below. A look at the offending object and a knowledge of
the underlying anatomy can be very useful in determining the extent of the
injury.

Any puncture wound more than a little deep should be watched carefully for
signs of infection, and considered for an immediate evacuation.

Impaled Object. It is unique to find a puncturing object still stuck into a human.
They usually pull it out as an instinctive reaction. And so you end up treating a
puncture wound. But the object may be still there because it broke off too short
to grab, or it is embedded too deeply, or the shape of the object caused it to
catch inside the flesh.

If you can get to a medical facility with relative ease, the object is probably
best padded to prevent movement, and the patient carried out of the woods. In
many cases there is nothing easy about getting to help. You can't heal with
something stuck in you, you can't prevent infection, and you aren't happy.

Removal of impaled objects in the backcountry is an oft-debated subject.
Yanking on an object can stimulate serious bleeding and damage underlying
structures. But they sometimes make evacuation very difficult. They can be
impossible to stabilize over rough terrain. Metal, like an ice axe, can suck a
significant amount of heat out of a cold patient.

If the object is through a cheek, or in any other way endangering the patient's airway, there is ample agreement on removing it carefully. If the object is
loosely embedded, removal is simple and beneficial to you and the patient. If the
object is in an extremity, removal is probably safe. Note the objects shape and
angle of entry, and remove accordingly. If the impaled object is large, and in a
body cavity (chest or abdomen), it is usually best to stabilize it in place as
snugly as possible, and evacuate with speed and great care.

There are no great answers here, but there are sound reasons for removing
an impaled object in the backcountry if the situation warrants.

Dressings and Bandages

The dressing is the primary covering of the open wound. It protects, reduces pain, absorbs exudates, and gives psychological relief. It should be sterile, non-adherent, porous, resistant to bacterial infiltration, and easy to use. Avoid confusion by purchasing a few pre-packaged dressings from your local drugstore. Buy an assortment of gauze pads, sponges, and band-aids. If a sterile dressing is unavailable, a piece of cloth can be sterilized by boiling. The formula for sterilization is a rolling boil for five minutes plus one minute more for every 1000 feet above sea level you are. This formula, once again, sterilizes, and should not be confused with disinfection, a simpler process. (Of course, for

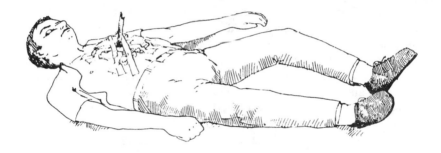

Figure 5–1
Stabilization of an impaled object.

minor open wounds, disinfection, just bringing the water to a rolling boil, might be enough. Consider the severity of the wound, and the time it will take to reach medical aid.)

Do not touch the sterile dressing except on the edges where it will not contact the wound. To provide adequate protection, the dressing should extend at least one inch past the borders of the wound.

The function of the bandage is to fix, protect, and further assist the dressing. It can be strips of clean cotton, elastic wraps, roller gauze, tape, or improvised out of anything you have. The usefulness of a bandage is handicapped by being too loose, and dangerous if applied tightly enough to restrict circulation. It should be put on snug, and checked often. Do not hide rings or anything that can cut off healthy blood flow if swelling occurs. If tape is used, it should be well away from the opening to keep the sticky stuff out of the wound. Tape should not be wrapped entirely around an extremity, which might make it into a tourniquet.

Tincture of benzoin applied to skin before taping makes the tape stick better for more long lasting results. Keep the benzoin out of the wound. It encourages infection, and hurts!

Specific Dressings and Bandages

Bandage strips. These self-adhering strips combine a dressing and a bandage (ie Bandaids). They come in various sizes, one inch x three inches usually doing the job, and are great for minor open wounds.

Butterfly bandages. The shape allows neat closure of gaping wounds. They can be improvised from tape, and semi-sterilized in the heat of a match along the middle section that will touch the wound. Special tape (ie. Steri-strips) can be used to close wounds.

Gauze pads. These sterile pads start in a one inch x one inch size and go on to huge dimensions. A 4x4 will meet most demands.

Sponges. These denser gauze pads work as a compress, absorbing more. A substitute is an individually-wrapped sanitary napkin. In an emergency, the sanitary napkin can be used for its intended purpose.

Roller gauze. These self-adhering rolls of gauze come in many widths, but four inches will usually work well, and is easy to handle. A bit of tape adds to the security, and their elasticity prevents them from cutting off circulation.

Elastic wraps. Although mostly used to support sprained joints, these wraps (ie. Ace) can compress a large wound while holding the dressing in place.

Adhesive tape. Again, several widths are available. The two-inch wide variety is a fine choice for the backcountry since it can be torn easily into a one-inch width if needed.

Triangular bandages. As the name implies, these are triangles of cloth. They can be created out of large bandannas with a simple fold. They can be used to tie on dressings, working well in difficult places like on the head. If large enough, they can be used as slings and swathes for the arm.

The Barehanded Principles: Wound Management

1. Take a close look at the injury.

2. Control the bleeding with direct pressure and elevation.

3. Clean your hands.

4. Clean the wound thoroughly.

5. Cover the wound with a sterile dressing and a bandage.

6. Splint a severely injured part.

7. Watch for signs of infection.

8. *Watch for signs of shock from blood loss.*
9. *Evacuate the patient if necessary.*

Burns

A burn, although common, is seldom a serious backcountry injury. They can be a nuisance, and they can lead to more significant problems if improperly treated. On occasion a burn can produce a life-threat.

Some chemicals, strong acids or alkalis mostly, can burn skin, but they are rarely carried beyond the roadhead. Electricity, in the form of lightning, is a potential hazard. A lightning strike usually gives us much more to be concerned about than the burns it might leave on our patient. Radiation from the sun is a very common cause of minor outdoor burning. But a thermal burn is the one that will most likely involve you, a burn produced by an extreme of temperature.

With any burn, there are three criteria determining the severity of the injury: depth, extent, and location.

First degree burns are superficial in depth, and do little to disrupt human tissue. The skin is irritated, red, painful. Second degree burns destroy some tissue. They are partial thickness burns, producing blisters that form minutes to hours after the initial contact with heat. Third degree burns extend through the full thickness of the skin, leaving charred remains of tissue. It is popular to point out the lack of pain in third degree burns due to the destruction of nerve endings in the skin, but the site is usually surrounded by second and first degree injuries that cause pain.

The extent, or size, of a burn is important. In adults the Rule of Nines can be applied to aid in determining the extent. The Rule says the head and neck are about 9% of the surface of a human, the arms are 9% each, legs are 18% each, the back of the torso is 18%, and the front of torso is another 18%. The missing one percent is found on the genitals. In infants and small children, the head is a significantly larger percentage of their body surface. Consider the head of infants to be 18% of their surface, the legs 13–14% each.

For smaller areas, the Rule of Hands can be used. This rule calls the area covered by your patient's hand approximately one percent of the total surface area of their body.

The location of the burn will help determine its severity. Injuries to the face and respiratory tract, the hands and feet, and the genitals can be critical.

Burns can be classified as either mild, moderate, or severe, and some disagreement exists over how to make that determination. Here is one way, but the most important determining factor will almost always be your patient: How are they doing?

Mild burns. Almost all first degree injuries can be considered mild, unless the area is extensive. Second degree burns that cover less than 15% of an adult, or

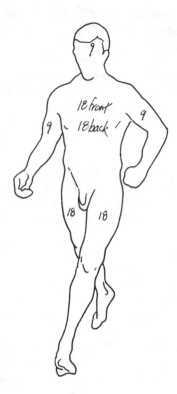

Figure 5–2
Rule of Nines.

10% of an infant or elder, are usually minor. And third degree burns that cover less than 3%, if no critical area is involved.

Moderate burns. First degree injuries covering more than three-fourths of an adult, or one-half of an infant are moderate. Or second degree burns over 15–25% of an adult, or 10–20% of an infant or elderly person. And third degree burns on 3–5% of a person when a critical area is not involved.

Severe burns. Critical burns would involve more than 25% of an adult if the injuries were second degree. Or second degree burns over 20% of an infant or elder. Or third degree burns over 5% of a body. Or third degree burns involving face, neck, hands, feet, or genitals. Or any burn complicating the airway. Or any third degree burn with underlying serious injuries such as fractures.

Emergency care of burns is initially the same despite the severity of the injury: Remove the victim from the source of the injury, and put out the fire. If they are in flames, smother the flames. Immediately flood the burned area in cold, clean water by pouring it on, by immersion, or by covering the area with a soaking wet, clean piece of cloth. Take off any burned clothing, and anything constricting in the area of the burn (rings, bracelets, watches). It is important to remember that hot skin and underlying tissues will continue to burn even after the source of the heat has been removed. Keep up the flood of water for at least ten minutes. Estimate the depth, extent, and involvement of critical areas.

First degree burns do not need any special treatment. Aloe, aloe gels, or a water-based moisturizing lotion (not oil-based) will help skin feel more comfortable as it heals.

Second degree burns should have the blisters covered with a sterile dressing to protect them from popping. An open blister presents a high risk of infection. If they do pop, treat the resulting open wound with the regimen of cleaning and protecting.

Third degree burns will probably get infected since the skin's ability to protect the victim has burned away. Cover the wound with a dry, sterile dressing and start planning your evacuation. The skin's waterproofness is gone, also, and a substantial flood of precious body fluids may escape producing "burn shock", a problem similar to extensive blood loss. Watch for it, and treat appropriately.

The greatest immediate threat to life is loss of an airway from burned and swollen air passages. Watch for hoarseness, difficulty breathing, a brassy cough or a cough producing sooty sputum, or any combination of the above. Look for burns on the face, and scorched facial hair. These people need to be rushed out to a hospital.

The Barehanded Principles:
Burns

1. *Remove victim from the source of the heat.*
2. *Put out the fire with copious amounts of cold water.*
3. *Remove burned clothing and restrictive jewelry and such.*
4. *Avoid breaking blisters open.*
5. *Cover burns with a dry, sterile dressing.*
6. *Watch for respiratory distress.*
7. *Watch for shock.*
8. *Evacuate if needed.*

Infection

On a worldwide basis, infection, the multiplication of harmful microorganisms in tissue of the body, is still the leading cause of death. In America we have become more civilized, and we die most often from the peaceful and sedentary problem of heart disease. We remain covered with microscopic life forms, especially on our skin, and in our mouths, throats, and intestines. Most of these organisms are harmless. If our internal defenses against disease are down, if we contact harmful organisms, or if an injury breaks us open, we might still develop a dangerous infection.

Our most common U.S. infections are colds and influenza, which we pass on directly or indirectly to each other, and label "contagious". The most common infection on our earth is malaria. Many infections are not contagious, such as those in the urinary tract, the appendix . . . and in wounds.

When the surface of a wound dries, a scab forms protecting the damaged area as healing goes on underneath. An unseen barrier develops on the inside of the body as well, sealing off the wound entirely. White blood cells attack the entrenched germs. Much of the contamination that migrates to the surface and drains out as white or faintly yellow pus is WBC's that died in the line of duty. Some of the contamination is dumped internally into the lymphatic system and carried to lymph nodes where it is picked up by our circulatory system and eventually cleaned out of the blood and excreted from our body. The wound wonderfully maintains itself. This complex body process is called inflammation. It looks a little red and swollen, feels a little warm and tender.

If the bacteria trapped in a wound are too abundant for the inflammation process to handle, infection will occur. The redness becomes redder, the warmth becomes heat, the swelling swells, and tissue begins to harden past the borders of the wound. These signs usually show up in 24–48 hours, but they can develop days after the accident. The pain may become great, and mobility of an extremity may be limited.

Wounds on the hand are the ones that most commonly become infected. Hands get less healthy circulation, are made of involved and overlapping tissue planes that trap bacteria easily, and are the most likely place for us to cut ourselves.

As infection spreads, lymph nodes can grow large and painful as they attempt to catch and kill the contamination, a condition known as lymphadenitis. The principal nodes are located in the elbows and knees, neck, groin, and along the mid-to-lower backbone. Less common in infected wounds, lymphangitis produces the red streaks that sometimes appear just under the skin. The streaks move from the wound toward the nearest lymph node as lymphatic vessels become inflamed. Should the infection reach the bloodstream, the result will likely be septicemia, sometimes called "blood poisoning", and the possibility of life-threatening shock (see SHOCK).

Some wounds are more susceptible to infection than others. Be especially careful of flesh torn open by the teeth of animals, the bites of cats and humans being especially prone to infection. Infection is likely to result from crushing injuries, burns that open the skin, and severe frostbite. Heavy foreign body contamination is responsible for a lot of problems, as with an unnoticed splinter of wood buried in a foot or hand.

Any infection, whatever the source, produces similar signs and symptoms once it spreads throughout a patient's system. The victim develops a fever with accompanying chills and malaise. Serious infections often cause headache, nausea, vomiting, or back pain.

Precious few places on earth are far from an antibiotic, but far out in the backcountry an infection might become a serious threat to life. Gas gangrene, for instance, the result of an anaerobic bacterium that produces rapidly spreading tissue destruction, can cause death in as little as 30 hours. Gangrenous wounds stir up an abundance of dark, foul-smelling pus.

If you suspect infection, evacuate your patient to a medical facility as soon as possible. In the meantime, provide rest, warmth, a soft or liquid diet, and a high fluid intake. Aspirin or acetaminophen may be given to reduce the fever. Stronger pain killers, if you have them, can temporarily ease the suffering. As you head for a doctor, keep track of the medications given. And keep tabs on the patient's temperature, if you have a thermometer.

You can aid your patient's struggle against an infected wound by opening the injury and scrubbing it clean. Soaking the wound in salty water as hot as the injured person can tolerate can be very helpful in the cleaning process. Hot compresses may also stimulate the wound to drain. If you tell your doctor about your adventures far from a hospital, you might even get a prescription for a general antibiotic. Be sure to get very specific written instructions about when and how to use the drug, and follow them.

The Barehanded Principles:
Infection

1. *Watch for a wound with increasing redness, swelling, pain, and pus.*
2. *Watch for fever and malaise.*
3. *Soak and scrub the wound clean.*
4. *As much as possible keep the patient rested and warm, with a soft diet and high fluid intake.*
5. *If available, give medications for fever and pain.*
6. *Evacuate.*

CHAPTER 6
INJURIES TO THE HEAD AND FACE

Introduction

Ice was forming on the rocky slope called Central Gully at the head of Huntington Ravine. It happens that way some Octobers on Mount Washington. A 20-year-old dayhiker moved off the trail seeking surer footing. She didn't find it. Slipping on a more technical section of the ravine, she tumbled about 100 feet, and finished in a free fall of 40 feet. Somewhere on the way down her face struck forcefully against stone. Her boyfriend ran for help.

The first responder arrived from the Appalachian Mountain Club approximately one hour later. He found her barely conscious, her eyes swollen shut, and cerebrospinal fluid (CSF) leaking from her nose. The responder radioed for immediate assistance, and realizing the possibilities, asked for a helicopter. We came on foot another hour further into the incident, and assessed her as critical.

With the patient packaged securely in a Stokes litter, we began the first of a series of six Z-drags that brought her eventually to the top of the ravine. It was more complicated to haul her up than down, but the nearest landing spot for the 'copter was a flat upper meadow.

Long after dark, she was lifted off for a quick flight to Boston. Extensive surgery was required, but she was able to return finally to a full and healthy life. The serious and often subtle complications of a severe head injury usually cause death in as little as four hours. Separating life and death for this young woman was early recognition of the seriousness of her accident.

Head Injury

The bulk of your brain is the cerebrum, the gray matter, the center of higher functions like thought and emotion. In the back of your head, beneath the cerebrum, is the cerebellum, where equilibrium and coordination are con-

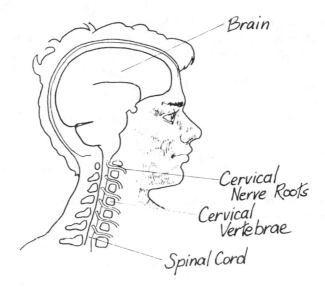

Figure 6–1
Interior arrangement of the brain and cervical spinal cord.

trolled. The brainstem grows out of the base of the brain and is responsible for vital vegetative functions, including circulation and respiration. Enclosing the brain, and the spinal cord, are three blood-rich layers of tissue called, collectively, the meninges. Their names, from the brain outward, are the pia mater, arachnoid, and dura mater. Cerebrospinal fluid, constantly filling the spaces between the meninges and bathing the brain and spinal cord, is a clear liquid protecting and feeding the central nervous system.

Your brain sits about one millimeter from the inside of your skull, comfortably in command of everything that goes on within you if the temperature, salt, water, blood sugar, and pressure stay balanced in your head. Head trauma ranges from simple scalp damage to severe brain damage. The severity is usually a result of the uncompromising structure of the skull (the cranium). If the brain starts to swell, it is squashed because there's no room up there for the swelling to take place.

Assessing Head Injury

For quick reference, head injuries can be loosely divided into four categories:

1) NO LOSS OF CONSCIOUSNESS means only an extremely rare chance of serious problems, despite the fact heavy bleeding and a huge goose-egg sized bump may accompany the injury. The brain has not been damaged.

2) MILD OR SHORT-TERM UNCONSCIOUSNESS tells that the victim's brain briefly contacted the inside of the cranium, and some transient loss of

function occurred. There is usually nothing to worry about. Keep in mind the victim may not be aware they have been unconscious. Ask witnesses, if possible. Watch for the tell-tale signs of increasing intracranial pressure (ICP), an announcement the brain is being threatened:

1. a headache that increases in intensity.
2. complaints of blurred vision or other visual disturbances.
3. a level of consciousness progressing from disoriented to irritable to combative to coma.
4. a heart rate slowing down and starting to bound.
5. noticeably irregular breathing, often progressing to deep and sighing breaths.
6. skin tending toward flushed and warm, especially in the face.
7. an increase in blood pressure.
8. pupils becoming unequal in size with loss of normal reaction to light.

3) LONG-TERM UNCONSCIOUSNESS is a serious warning that the ICP is on the rise. The problem may be a bruise to the brain, or a tear in the blood vessels of the meninges, or a laceration of the brain itself. The tough dura mater may be clinging to the inside of the cranium, with blood collecting between the dura and the bone (an epidural hematoma). A subdural hematoma is blood pooling between the dura and the brain. The blood can gather over hours, or weeks, increasing the pressure until death results.

4) OBVIOUS HEAD INJURIES include a depressed spot where the skull is fractured, visible fracture lines where a portion of the scalp has been torn away, black-and-blue around swollen eyes (Raccoon eyes), black-and-blue behind and below the ears (Battle's sign), and blood or clear cerebrospinal fluid (or both mixed) leaking from the nose or ears. Seizures are common.

Treating Head Injuries

To be safe, don't wait for the danger signals. Evacuate to professional medical attention anyone who has been forcefully knocked unconscious, even if they appear OK initially.

Maxim: Evacuate Anyone Knocked Unconscious.

They can walk out if there are no obvious signs of injury. If there is a strong suspicion of injury, move them gently to prevent possible damage to their cervical spine, which is often at risk from a severe blow to the head (see SPINAL CORD INJURY MANAGEMENT). They need to have their entire spine immobilized. In the meantime, keep them lying down. If they must be left alone for any reason, roll them carefully onto their side (the recovery position), to ensure an airway. Deeply unconscious people lose muscle tone, including their tongue which can fall back over their airway. Head injured people like to vomit, sometimes on a regular basis, and aspirated vomitus (vomit sucked into the lungs) usually causes death. Keep them lying down, on a slope if you can, with their

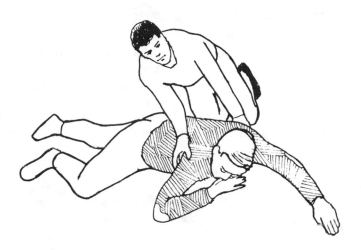

Figure 6–2
Recovery position to maintain an open airway.

head slightly uphill. You may be able to reduce the swelling rate of the brain with gravity's aid.

Once in a hospital, even the seriously head injured patient has a great chance of survival. Oxygen therapy, drug therapy, and surgical intervention are available. That's why they keep the patient awake, or arouse them regularly. If arousal is impossible, it is time for radical procedures. In a backcountry situation, let your patient sleep if they want to. In sleep, the brain will have the best chance of controlling its own swelling.

Deep in the wilderness, a serious head injury is a serious threat to life. Given the time and distance from help, you may be called upon to make a tough decision. Should you carry them out the best you can? Should you go for assistance? There are no absolute answers! If your patient is showing signs of improvement after 48 hours, their prognosis is very good.

The Barehanded Principles: Head Injury

1. Maintain an airway.

2. Keep them on their side, if necessary.

3. Evacuate all suspects of increasing ICP.

4. Let them sleep if they want to.
5. Treat for possible cervical spine injury.

Injuries to the Face

The greatest danger from an injury to the face, whether it be soft tissue damage or fractures of the facial bones, is obstruction of the patient's airway. Management of any face injury needs to include a careful watch to keep the airway clear, and the assumption that their cervical spine is damaged until proven otherwise. This might mean carefully arranging your patient on their side if they're unconscious to let blood flow out of the airway instead of down their windpipe.

The Ear

That flap of flesh, the external ear, directs sound down a canal to the eardrum, the tympanic membrane, where the vibrations are transmitted to the three little bones of the middle ear. A tube leads from the middle ear to the nose, balancing the pressure and allowing you the interesting pastime of pinching your nose and blowing to make your ears pop as the pressure changes. The little bones pass the vibrations on to the snail-shaped cochlea of the inner ear, which breaks the sound up before sending it along nerve pathways to the brain for decoding.

An injury to the ear will probably be external damage that is obvious and treated as any soft tissue injury is handled, or a ruptured eardrum. Damage to the eardrum can be caused by a blow to the side of the head, a change in pressure while diving underwater, a nearby explosion (possible in a lightning strike), or a foreign object stuck up the ear canal. The patient will complain of pain, ringing or whistling in their ear, or loss of hearing, and maybe a loss of coordination (an upsetting phenomenon called vertigo).

If there's a possibility of a related head injury, DO NOT TRY TO STOP THE FLOW OF BLOOD FROM THE INSIDE OF AN INJURED EAR. They may be relieving their own increasing intracranial pressure. Cover their ear with bulky sterile dressings, preventing further contamination without stopping the flow. Do not stick an instrument into the ear, or try to remove a lodged foreign body. Evacuation to the care of a physician is necessary.

The Eye

The eyeball is truly round, but only a small slice shows to the outside world. A jelly-like fluid called vitreous humor fills the ball. A bulge, the cornea, sits on the front of the eyeball and is filled with salty fluid called aqueous humor. Between the bulge and the ball lies the lens. Over the lens is a special muscle, the iris, that has an adjustable opening, the pupil. Working together, they focus images on a layer of sensitive cells, the retina, covering the back of the eye. Translated into electrical signals and carried by the optic nerves from each eye to the back of the brain, the image is decoded into thought. Since the images are translated from the back of the brain, sometimes a blow to the back of the head causes visual disturbances.

Nature has determined to protect our eyes in several ways. The outside of the ball, except over the cornea, is covered with a tough membrane called the sclera, the "white" of the eye. A thin, mucous membrane, the conjunctiva, covers the exposed part of the eye and the inner side of the eyelid. Together these see-through "skins" are much hardier than the skin that covers the rest of our bodies. Lacrimal (tear) glands keep the eye moist, washing out most of the dust and debris. The eyelids add protection and help keep the surface of the eye clean when you blink. A bony socket, the orbit, surrounds everything and forms a protective shield. It is lined with fatty "shock absorbers", a final barrier against physical abuse. Still, it is possible to injure the eye.

Foreign Matter in the Eye

The most common problem is when something is in your eye that doesn't belong: debris, hair, insects. The discomfort can be enormous, but usually the victim's own tearing mechanism will wash the eye clean before any serious damage occurs. Healthy first aid is simply to avoid rubbing the eye and immediately washing it out with a lot of clean water.

Lie the patient down while a steady stream of water is poured on the bridge of the nose. Rapid blinking encourages the flushing process.

There is nothing harmful about removing large chunks of debris from an eye, as long as force is never used. If the matter does not come loose with the aid of a soft tissue or additional rinsing, leave it alone, cover the eye with a folded gauze pad or sterile eye patch, and get to a doctor. Also, never try to remove anything stuck to the surface of the cornea.

Occasionally the eye will feel irritated after the matter has been removed, making it painful to blink. Most likely, the eye has suffered an abrasion. Rinse the eye again, and if still uncomfortable, patch it shut. Take an anti-inflammatory analgesic like ibuprofen. Do not apply a topical anesthetic without a physician's advice. Often they can slow healing, inhibit your eye's protective reflexes, and cause further damage to the tissue. For irritation that persists for 24 hours, head for a doctor.

Contusions

The classic "black eye" is a result of rapid swelling and discoloration following a blow. The whites may also turn an alarming red. But don't worry. A cold compress will reduce the pain and swelling. Within 12 to 24 hours the eye will look relatively normal in size. It can take a week to 10 days for the "black" to fade.

Reasons to see a doctor after a punch in the eye include persistent blurred vision, double vision, extraordinary sensitivity to light, and discharge of something other than tears.

Punctures

An eyeball impaled with a sharp object is a serious injury. If the object is still there, do not try to remove it. Keep the patient lying down to prevent gravity from pulling the critically important vitreous humor out.

Stabilizing what has pierced the eye is necessary. One way to do this is to make a "donut" out of a rolled hankerchief or triangular bandage. Place it gently around the eye, adding a cup over the donut so nothing can catch or jar the object. Tape it all securely, and patch the other eye shut as well. If the good eye looks around nervously, the bad eye will try to follow it, possibly causing more damage. Carry the patient to a hospital.

Lacerations of the Eyelid

A cut in the lid produces a lot of blood. Relax, and check the eyeball for damage. If it has been cut, the patient must be kept still and lying down, with both eyes patched. Otherwise, cover the wound with a light, sterile dressing. Although the slice may be quite small, a scar on the eyelid can be a discomfort for the rest of your life. Doctors can stitch the wound neatly with little or no noticeable scarring.

The Nose

Nose injuries usually produce one or two similar manifestations: pain and blood. Keep the patient sitting up and leaning slightly forward, if possible, to prevent blood from entering their airway. If blood is visibly running out, pinch the nostrils closed, using direct pressure to promote clotting. Try to prevent your patient from moving around for about a half hour after the bleeding stops, to give clotting a chance to complete. Instruct your patient to please restrain from nose picking, sneezing, and bending over and straining for the next couple of days.

A nose bleed (epistaxis) is almost always anterior. A few, especially in people with chronic high blood pressure, may be posterior. The blood runs down the throat, and the patient may require a doctor's care to stop the bleeding.

Susceptible people are encouraged to have nose bleeds by dry weather. Applications of an ointment inside the nose can reduce the dryness, and prevent bleeds. The same stuff you use on dry lips will work if gently applied to the inside of the nose once or twice a day.

To avoid the possibility of serious damage, an object securely wedged inside a nose should be left in place until a physician can remove it.

Rapid swelling often makes it difficult to make an assessment of a broken nose. If you aren't sure, give the patient painkillers and apply cold packs for 20 to 30 minutes, three or four times a day. If their level of discomfort is acceptable to them, it is OK to let them stay in the backcountry. When the nose is obviously broken, the same treatment is advisable, but consider evacuation to a medical facility as well. Your patient may wish to have a bit of surgery done so they'll eventually look the same. There is no rush. The surgery will be just as successful if a week goes by first. In fact, some surgeons like to have the patient wait until the swelling goes down, since it's easier to tell where to realign the nose.

The Mouth

A profuseness of blood vessels in the mouth leads to an abundance of bleeding from even very trivial wounds to that area. Active bleeding from mouth trauma almost always stops on its own, and immediate care of the patient should center on maintaining an open airway. If they have been knocked unconscious, airway maintenance might necessitate logrolling the patient onto their side while keeping alignment of the cervical spine. If they're conscious and you suspect no c-spine injury, keep them sitting up and leaning slightly forward.

Mouth lacerations tend to look horrible for the first couple of days, but they also tend to heal nicely with little care. The patient should rinse their mouth with water every two or three hours and after every meal until the wound is completely closed.

If the wound gapes open significantly, the patient should be evacuated from the backcountry for stitches, especially if the lips are involved. Gaping wounds to the mouth and lips that heal puckered are unsightly, in the way, and difficult to repair once they heal that way.

(See DENTAL EMERGENCIES for the treatment of injuries involving the teeth.)

CHAPTER 7
CHEST INJURIES

Introduction

Leaving the groomed slope for the trees was not her idea. She intended to curve gracefully down to the lodge on one final run. But a combination of fatigue and ice sent her off route and into a high-speed collision with a sturdy white pine.

Labored breathing claimed the immediate attention of her rescuers. It was difficult for her to find a position of comfort, and she squirmed in the snow, moaning vigorously. A quick secondary assessment showed an angulated upper left arm and remarkable pain in the pelvis. Her vital signs indicated she was considering going into the progressive stages of shock.

The sled held a full spineboard, and even though it was well padded, she complained of the pain of being stabilized on it. Her breathing decreased in quality, and increased in rate. Her anxiety increased.

At the hut supplemental oxygen was started at a high flow, but her level of consciousness continued to decrease on the long ski out. Her short, gasping respirations could be heard above the sound of skis cutting the hard snow. At the ambulance she responded only to painful stimulus.

The hospital's x-rays revealed neat fractures of the arm and pelvis, easily treated. Of more critical concern was the splinters of bone from three shattered ribs on the left side. At least one piece of bone had punctured a lung. Air leaking out of the lung was filling her chest cavity and making it more and more difficult to adequately exchange oxygen. Her full recovery would have been impossible without rapid surgical intervention.

How We Breathe

Our breathing apparatus is composed partly of twelve pairs of ribs. All are firmly attached in back to vertebrae, and the top ten adhere to the sternum in

44

front. The last two float freely low in the chest. A dome-shaped muscle, the diaphragm, is curved along the lower line of the ribs, separating the lungs and heart from the lower organs. The lungs are five spongy lobes, three on our right and two on our left, made of thousands of tiny grape-like clusters of alveoli bunched at the end of bronchioles. A tough membrane, the visceral pleura, surrounds each lung. A continuation of the membrane, the parietal pleura, lines the inner chest wall. Between the two membranes is a *potential* space, the pleural cavity, which should remain potential because the lungs are designed to stick to the inside of the rib cage.

On inspiration the muscles between the ribs flex and the ribs are pulled upward. The diaphragm flexes and thus flattens, pulling downward. The lungs slide along the inner chest wall, but are forced open since a fluid keeps them from pulling away. Negative pressure is created inside the chest, and air rushes in through the nose or mouth, down the windpipe to where it divides into a right and left bronchus, into bronchioles of ever-decreasing size until it reaches a sac of alveoli. At the alveoli oxygen in the air is exchanged for carbon dioxide in the blood, and life goes on. Inspiration is the active phase of breathing.

On expiration the muscles relax, returning to their normal position. The elastic tissues of the lungs are pulled back to their original position. Air is pushed out. Expiration is the passive phase of breathing.

Chest Injuries

An injury to the chest can be closed, the damage done inside the patient without anything penetrating the integrity of the chest wall. The injury can be open, the result of the forceful entry of an object.

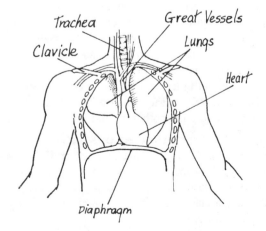

Figure 7-1
Interior arrangement of the chest.

Fractured Ribs

Breaking a rib or two is the most common injury to the chest, and the fifth to the tenth ribs are most commonly involved. The first four are protected by the shoulder, and the freedom in front enjoyed by the last two allow them to absorb more of a blow.

Patients complain of localized pain after receiving a direct hit on the chest wall. They like to sit hunched forward, their arms protectively holding the injury, and breathing shallowly to ease the discomfort.

The pain may be great, but if the fracture is simple and uncomplicated the patient may safely choose to stay in the backcountry. Whether they stay or go, a sling and swathe on the injured side often eases the discomfort by supporting the muscles that are spasming and causing the pain. Any activity aggravating the injury should be avoided, and it is best to see a physician once one is available.

Pneumothorax

Air (pneumo) enters the chest (thorax), which sounds like a healthy occurrence except this air is entering the pleural space from a tear in the lung made by a complicated fractured rib. The vacuum between the visceral and parietal pleura is destroyed, and, as air collects in the no-longer-potential space, the lung eventually collapses. The patient has more and more difficulty breathing. Their hearts tend to speed up as their level of anxiety rises. Suspect this injury in anyone who has received a blow to the chest and demonstrates increasing respiratory distress.

This patient needs a physician as soon as possible. It will be best if they are carried. Walking will increase their need for oxygen and complicate their breathing. They will usually travel easiest in a semi-sitting position.

Tension Pneumothorax

Excessive air pressure in the pleural cavity makes it impossible for the patient to adequately breathe. Their heart, trachea (windpipe), and large blood vessels of the chest are pushed toward the uninjured side by the increasing pressure. The injured side of the chest becomes rigid and distended. Subcutaneous emphysema, air forced up through the skin, may give the patient a bloated appearance. The bloated skin will crackle if you push on it. Watch for the signs and symptoms of shock.

Death results unless a qualified person opens an appropriate hole in the injured chest to relieve the pressure. It is best to try to anticipate the development of a tension pneumothorax, and start an evacuation as soon as possible.

Spontaneous Pneumothorax

Someone with emphysema or another lung disease, or a person who is otherwise predisposed, may develop a pneumothorax spontaneously, without trauma to the chest. A lung suddenly ruptures, allowing air into the pleural space. Sudden stabbing chest pain and increasing difficulty breathing should create suspicion of this condition.

Hemothorax

Damage to the chest may result in an accumulation of blood in the chest cavity. A hemothorax often occurs simultaneously with a pneumothorax. The blood collects in the lower area of the lung, and may be difficult if not impossible to assess. The signs and symptoms will be the same as with a pneumothorax, and management of the patient will be the same.

Contusions

A blow to the chest may bruise the heart or lungs. The result may be chest pain and the signs and symptoms of shock with disturbances in the rhythm of the heart (bruised heart) or respiratory distress with a cough that produces blood (lung bruise). General principles for treating a chest injury should be followed. If the patient feels like coughing up blood, encourage them to do so, which helps keep their lungs free of excess fluid.

Pericardial Tamponade

Around the heart lies a tough membrane called the pericardial sac (or pericardium). Trauma to the chest may cause a tear in the heart, allowing blood to leak out and fill the sac. The heart is compressed and each succeeding beat is less efficient than the one before. The heart beats faster and weaker as the pressure on it increases. The patient grows increasingly anxious and short of breath. It is not easy to assess pericardial tamponade. If the blood pressure can be checked a drop in systolic will be noted with a corresponding slight rise in diastolic. As with any serious chest injury, the patient needs surgical intervention to live.

Flail

A flail is a free-floating piece of chest wall created when three or more adjacent ribs are broken in two or more places. The result is paradoxical respirations, the free piece moving in opposition to the rest of the chest. Pain is great, and difficulty breathing is extreme. As with any suspicion of serious chest injury, take a look at the patient's chest. Here you will see the paradoxical movement, maybe not at first when muscle spasms hold the flail in place, but certainly later as the muscles fatigue. Asking the patient to inhale deeply will allow you to assess pain and deformity early.

A flail creates a dire emergency. Oxygen demands cannot be met by the inadequate respirations, and respiratory failure is not far away.

Immediate management is the only hope of saving this patient. If they are unconscious, roll them on to their injured side, hoping to reduce some of the movement of the flail. This "recovery position" helps keep their airway open as well. If they are conscious, hold the flail in place with your hand until you can make a pad to fit the flail. Folded clothing or a cut-to-fit piece of sleeping pad will work. Tape the pad securely in place, but do not run the strips of tape completely around the chest, which reduces the ability to breathe. Run the tape well past the pad, and run some strips vertically and some horizontally. Tincture of benzoin, if you remembered to put some in your first aid kit, helps hold the tape to sweaty skin. If the respiratory distress becomes acute, start positive pressure ventilations (pinch their nose, seal your mouth over theirs, and breath for them every time they make the effort to breathe). If they stop living, do CPR. Evacuation to a medical facility is, of course, essential.

Sucking Chest Wound

The sucking noise is made by air being pulled into the pleural space by the pressure of inhalation because something from the outside has penetrated the chest wall. This can happen by being shot or stabbed. Sometimes called an open pneumothorax, the air sucked in through the wound is useless, but it takes up the space needed for normal breathing to happen. Air flows in and out of the hole instead of in and out of the normal air passages. The patient rapidly asphyxiates.

Immediately seal the wound with your hand. As soon as possible, make a more permanent cover for the hole with a material that lets no air or water through, like a plastic bag. Tape it securely in place. Keep the patient in the position of comfort they chose (which is usually a semi-sitting position). During evacuation, monitor them closely for increasing respiratory distress, a sign they are developing a tension pneumothorax, possible now since you closed their chest. If it happens, tear off the seal and let the air out of the chest. Clotting may make this difficult without pulling away the clotted blood. With the pressure relieved, replace the seal. (Some rescuers claim success by taping the original seal in place on three sides only, allowing the tension to self-release.) Positive pressure ventilations may be necessary. CPR should be initiated immediately if the patient goes into cardiac arrest.

Impaled Object

If the object puncturing a chest is still there, every attempt should be made to leave it there. Great care should be taken to immobilize it in place since even slight movement may result in further internal damage. Lots of bulky padding will be helpful, and extreme carefulness in evacuation.

Truthfully, it is not always possible to give a victim ideal treatment. Some people will insist on impaling themselves on the most awkward objects (like stout limbs of trees). Keeping the principles of chest injury management in mind, you may be called upon to do your creative best.

The Barehanded Principles:
Chest Injury Management

1. *Maintain an open airway.*
2. *Let conscious patients assume the position of most comfort.*
3. *If respirations are difficult, take a look at the chest.*

4. *Treat the injury you find: sling and swathe the arm on the side of a fractured rib, stabilize the flail, plug sucking chest wound, immobilize the impaled object.*
5. *Assist with breathing, if necessary.*
6. *Carry out all but the most trivial chest injuries.*
7. *Encourage an occasional deep breath and the coughing up of any accumulating fluids.*

CHAPTER 8
ABDOMINAL INJURIES

The call from the lodge said a skier was complaining of severe abdominal pain. He was curled into a comfortable looking chair, but he was looking uncomfortable. A peek at the area where he said the pain was greatest revealed a bruise over his upper left abdomen, just below the ribs. His breaths came rapid and shallow, his heart raced. He was pale and pasty.

To the question "What happened?", he described gaining too much air on a jump, losing control, and landing forcefully on his left side. The wind whooshed out of him. He was lean and fit, and, pulling himself together, skied on down for a cup of coffee and the slow onset of shock.

Within two hours of arriving at the local hospital, his ruptured spleen lay in a basin on an operating room table. Without the operation, the same two hours would have been the rest of his life.

Packed into the region between our diaphragm and our groin are many important parts that can be crushed by the force of blunt trauma creating a closed injury, or torn by penetrating objects creating an open injury. Some of the parts are solid (pancreas, liver, kidneys, spleen) and mostly tucked under the rib cage for more protection, and some are hollow (stomach, intestines, gallbladder, urinary bladder, female reproductive organs). The lining of the abdominal cavity is a membrane called the peritoneum. Officially, the cavity has three parts: the abdomen, the retroperitoneum (the space behind the peritoneum where the kidneys and pancreas sit), and the subperitoneum (or pelvic region). Your treatment will not be hindered if you simply think of it all as "the abdomen". But it will help in your assessment to know generally where the organs are supposed to be.

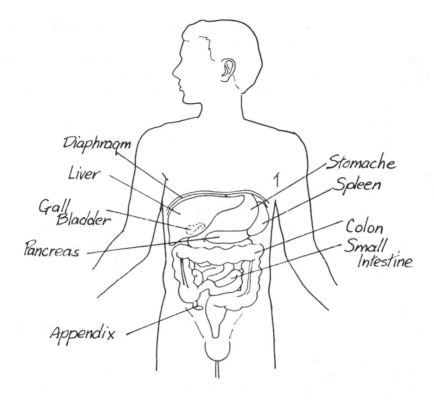

Figure 8-1
Interior arrangement of the abdomen.

Blunt Trauma

The victim of a severe blow to the abdomen needs to have an adequate history taken since what has taken place inside is not very obvious. What hit him? How fast was it going? Where is the pain? Does anything *provoke* the pain? What is its *quality?* (Ask him to rate it from one-to-ten). Has it begun to *radiate* from the original pain site? Evaluate the *severity*. What *time* did the pain start? These are the PQRST questions of patient assessment.

Trauma tearing open internal organs releases whatever the organ held. For hollow organs it may be things like stomach acid, digested food, or bacteria. Hollow organs contents are highly irritating. They cause an inflammatory reaction in the peritoneum called peritonitis. Pain may be described as sharp, stabbing, or burning, and it increases and spreads throughout the abdomen. Pulse and respirations quicken. The muscles of the abdomen become increasingly rigid and distended. Your ear placed against the patient's abdomen, periodically, reveals a decrease in the gurgles and rumbles of normal bowel activity as the intestines become paralyzed. The patient will lie very still on his back or side but demand flexion of his knees to take pressure off his abdominal muscles. Pain is provoked by movement and any attempt to straighten the legs.

Solid organs bleed when ruptured. Since blood is less irritating than hollow organ contents the signs and symptoms of peritonitis may not appear. The signs and symptoms of shock should appear. You should also see increasing rigidity, distention, and pain in the abdomen, and possibly the loss of bowel sounds.

With any abdominal injury anticipate nausea and vomiting. Over time, blood may appear in the vomit, urine, or stool of the patient. He may develop a fever.

Penetrating Injuries

In the backcountry the penetrating object could be a knife or gun, an ice axe or a ski pole. The immediate seriousness of the injury is determined by what got damaged inside. Over time the risk of infection is very high.

General assessment of the patient is the same as with a closed injury. Treatment will vary somewhat depending on the soft tissue involvement.

Treatment

Patients with abdominal injuries should be kept in the position of comfort they chose, and kept warm. If you are involved in their evacuation, comfort and warmth should be extended to them during the carry. Monitor them for the vomit that commonly appears, and be sure it is kept out of their airway. Nothing should be given to them by mouth. (On an extended evacuation, something over 24 hours, occasional small sips of cold water may be necessary to prevent dehydration.)

In an open injury, external bleeding can be controlled with direct pressure. The wound should be cleaned and bandaged as usual. If organs are protruding (called an evisceration), do not try to wash them, and do not try to push them back inside. Cover them with a sterile dressing followed by an occlusive (airtight, waterproof) covering. If freezing is not a concern, moistening the sterile dressing can be helpful. When an object is impaled in the abdominal cavity, it should be immobilized, held in place with soft bulky padding and tape or rolled bandages, to prevent further injury.

Abdominal injuries need rapid evacuation. Often surgical intervention is all that will eventually prevent their untimely death.

The Barehanded Principles: Abdominal Injuries

1. *Keep the patient in his chosen position of comfort, and keep him warm.*
2. *Give the patient nothing by mouth.*

3. *Watch for vomiting, and maintain the airway.*
4. *Control obvious bleeding, and manage open wounds.*
5. *Cover eviscerated organs with sterile and occlusive dressings.*
6. *Stabilize impaled objects in place.*
7. *Evacuate the patient as soon as possible, in a position of comfort, being careful to avoid undue movement.*

CHAPTER 9
STRAINS AND SPRAINS

David chose to ride his mountain bike along the old cross-country ski trail. It was too good a day to stay inside. Spring green blurred the distance in a vernal mist. The snow was gone, and the leaves were slickly matted to the ground after their recent burial. There's a pitch where the creek jumps off a rock face and you have to portage your bike, but otherwise the ride is long and relatively flat, and just right for getting out quick. David was alone again, as he often preferred.

Tired, and a bit out of shape, he pushed too hard on the return run to asphalt. A half-mile out, where the trail corners, he lost traction in a patch of wet leaves. Throwing his right leg out for support, his ankle rolled and exploded in pain. He tried to stop the ground from coming up so fast, but something popped in his right wrist. For a few minutes he lay on the soggy carpet, wishing his ankle belonged to someone else.

The most immediate question is: HOW SERIOUS IS IT? Probing around the ankle with his healthy hand, David found nothing saying broken bone, no unusual movement, no numbness or tingling in his foot, no exceptional feeling of cold, nothing to distinguish one ankle from the other, except the pain. Strain, sprain, or fracture, all serious musculoskeletal injuries have one thing in common—they are too painful to use. Intuitively, David trusted his ankle. He tried it, and it still worked. And so did his wrist. He rode out slowly, packed the bike on top of his car, and drove the ten miles home for a hot shower and dinner.

Next morning, the swelling and discoloration in his ankle would've made his own mother turn away. His wrist was sore but functional. Mismanagement had turned a minor injury into a big problem. A couple of days ago, over two years since the accident, David sat by my fire chatting. He complained of the soreness in his right ankle.

Strains

A fracture (a break in a bone) needs a splint, a trip to an emergency room, an X-ray, a cast, and a few weeks to months to heal permanently. A strain is a stretch in a muscle, similar to what weightlifters do on purpose. What happened, the mechanism of injury, the forces involved, give big clues as to whether you have a strain or a break.

Strains can be debilitating, especially in the lower back. Should you treat them with heat or cold? If the pain came on suddenly, cold should be applied for 20 to 30 minutes, several times a day, for the first 48 hours. If the pain grew gradually, heat usually works best. After two days, heat is best in most cases. The muscle can be used within the limits of pain. In other words, if it hurts don't do it!

Reasons to evacuate your patient for medical attention include: 1) the pain (or numbness) begins to radiate all the way down an arm or leg, 2) the pain remains strong even when the muscles are at rest, 3) the pain started as a result of illness, and 4) the pain came on sharply after a fall from a height or a sudden jolting stop.

Sprains

A sprain is damage to a joint, the mechanism similar to the movement producing dislocations, but with less force. Sprains involve the ligaments holding a joint together, and can vary in degree from simple over-stretching to complete tears. Unlike fractures that mend strong, and strains that heal well, a sprain is likely to bother you for the rest of your life, especially if you treat it improperly. What's really unfortunate about these injuries is that they don't hurt as much as they should. Pain would encourage us to act sensibly. Sensible action has three stages: First Aid, Rest, and Retraining.

Our first response is critical. Every minute RICE is delayed can add an hour to healing. RICE is an acronym for Rest, Ice, Compression, and Elevation. Stay off the injury (Rest) for the first half hour while you reduce its temperature (Ice) as much as possible without freezing. Crushed ice is best. It conforms to the shape of the anatomy involved. Do not put the ice directly on skin since that could produce a cold injury. Wrap the ice with a shirt or sock. Without ice, soak in cold water, or carry chemical coldpacks in your first aid kit, or (during warm months) submerge the joint in a wet T-shirt, or something else of cotton, and let evaporation cool the damaged area. Compression requires an elastic bandage (ie. Ace). Placing spare socks around the injury beneath the Ace keeps the compression more uniform. Wrap it snug, but watch it carefully for loss of circulation, the tingling, numbness, and pain, due to over-aggressive compression. Elevation refers to keeping the injury higher than the patient's heart. After RICE-ing, let rewarming happen for 10–15 minutes before trying to use the joint, to prevent further damage the ice-induced anaesthesia might allow. Monitor the amount of swelling and discoloration.

The goal of RICE is limiting swelling. The more the injury swells, the less you move it. The less you move, the quicker the muscles deteriorate. The faster the muscle atrophies, the longer it takes to heal. Over the next 48 hours, use the injury as little as possible, keep the compression on, repeat the icing regularly (three or four times per day).

As soon as the swelling stops getting worse, start exercising the joint. Wiggle it gently, spell the alphabet in the air with your toe. Add mild heat to loosen the stiffness, but warm up the water no hotter than a few degrees above body temperature. If swelling starts to increase, go back to cold. But keep up the exercising as much as pain will allow. You are increasing circulation to carry off the excess fluid and dead cells surrounding the injury, and smoothing out the fibers of the ligaments, and strengthening the muscles. You are speeding healing.

Even a mild sprain will take two months to heal solidly. You may be comfortable in one week, and feeling marvelous in two. But do not be fooled. Exercise your injured joint aggressively, but do not push it past the point of pain. If you are worse the next day, retreat, gather your strength, and push forward with more gentleness.

How do you know when you're well? Test your joints independently of each other, increasing the pressure on them slowly. Is your balance the same? Is your strength the same? Does the injured side hurt while the healthy side doesn't? Hop a few times on that sprained ankle. If you can't, you aren't completely healed. When your strength and pain responses are bilaterally equal for approximately ten repetitions of the same movement, you are ready to increase your training schedule.

Shoulders, elbows, wrists, fingers, knees, ankles, toes can all be sprained, and the supporting muscles can be strained. The principles for treatment don't change with the body part: a RICE period, a rest period, a retraining period. But stretching and strengthening should be specific to the injured area.

Evacuation

With most injuries, the patient is all the questions and all the answers. With minor musculoskeletal injuries this is very true. Can they bear the workload necessary to stay in the backcountry? Can they bear the pressure of the group if they can't keep up? Are they having fun? Do you think they are substantially increasing the risk to themselves or the group? If the patient is mobile, the final decision about whether to evacuate or not will depend on the many parts that make the whole picture.

The Barehanded Principles:
Strains and Sprains

*1. Rest, Ice, Compress, and Elevate the injury as
   soon as possible.*

2. Let it rewarm for 10 to 15 minutes.

3. *Test the injury for seriousness? usability?*
4. *If they stay in the backcountry, repeat RICE-ing 3 to 4 times/day for at least 48 hours.*
5. *If the patient is unsafe, unwell, or unhappy, evacuate them.*

CHAPTER 10
FRACTURES

Introduction

Miriam moved down the hard-packed snow slope cautiously. A fierce June sun burned overhead. Her crampons took a solid bite of the glacier, but it was her first time descending steep terrain. Miriam was afraid, wishing she had taken the leader's advice and stayed close to camp. Slipping out on her own, she had found going up easy, and climbed much higher than her original intention.

At least the others could see her. Crowded together near the colorful nylon village of tents, they waved. Their voices of encouragement drifted up muffled and unintelligible. Miriam lifted her ice axe to wave back. It was a mistake. Her tenuous balance gave out under the added stress, and she fell to her backside, gaining speed rapidly as she flailed for a brake. By the time she hit the exposed rocks at the end of the glacier, she was moving with enough force to snap her right femur, the large bone of her thigh.

The pain was intense, and swelling started almost immediately. Group members were at her side in moments, and were required to pull traction on her leg. Traction eased the pain, but the slightest movement ripped screams from Miriam. It was impossible to move her more than a few feet.

Before sending for help, a complete assessment was made, checking for any injuries the pain of the broken femur might be masking. A note was written, giving details of who, what, when, and where. The note was attached to a marked map, and three well-equipped, strong hikers were sent to request a helicopter. It was fourteen miles to the nearest road.

While the three "runners" were still preparing to leave, the leader rigged an improvised traction splint for Miriam's leg. He sliced the floor of a free-standing tent from end to end and set it up over her. With difficulty, they were able to get her onto an ensolite pad, off the cold surface of the mountain. For two uncomfortable days, the group stayed close to the patient, helping her maintain body warmth, giving her food and water, assisting her as she eliminated her body's wastes.

The care Miriam received on the mountain kept her leg intact. Surgical placement of a rod down the inside of her bone was required to complete full healing. But the story could have ended in permanent loss of function, or loss of leg.

Assessment

Fractures of bones in the arms and legs make up a large percentage of injuries in the backcountry. Sometimes the assessment is simple. Bones protrude through the skin, or angulations in the bones create joints where there aren't supposed to be any. Without the obvious, and without a radiographic picture of the bones, the rescuer can base the assessment of a fracture on common sense and a good LAF at the injury.

The L of LAF stands for Look. Remove or cut away clothing carefully and take a look at the site of the injury. (In cold weather this cutting away should be kept to a minimum.) Is there discoloration and swelling? Can the patient move the injury or do they guard it carefully? Compare the injured side to the uninjured side. Does it LOOK broken?

The A of LAF stands for ASK. Ask the patient to rate their pain. Does the patient think they're broken? Did they feel anything break? How did the injury occur? High speed impacts cause more breaks than low speed impacts. Torqued bones break more often than straight on impacts. How willing is the patient to *use* the injury?

The F stands for FEEL. Does the area of the injury feel rigid with spasms of the surrounding muscle? Does it feel unstable? Is there "point tenderness", a place on the bone that hurts noticeably more when you touch that spot? Check for Circulation, Sensation, and Motion (CSM) beyond the site of the injury. Loss of a pulse, numbness, tingling, and inability to move are signs of loss of adequate blood flow, the most immediately serious complication of a fracture.

Maxim: When in Doubt, Splint!
Splinting

The goal of a healthy splint is to immobilize the damaged bone(s), preventing further injury and increasing patient comfort until a medical facility can be reached. To do this best, the splint needs to be made of 1) something well-padded next to the patient and, 2) something rigid for additional support. Some fractures require 3) immobilization of the joints above and below the fractured bone to properly splint the injury.

Splints should immobilize the injured bone in the position of function, or as close to the position of function as possible. Functional position means legs almost straight with a slight flexion at the knee, feet at 90 degrees to legs, arms in 90 degrees of flexion, wrists straight, and fingers flexed into a functional curve. A spine, including neck and pelvis, should be splinted straight.

In choosing materials for splinting you are only limited by your imagination. For padding there are sleeping bags, ensolite pads (which you can cut to fit the problem), extra clothing, even soft debris from the forest floor stuffed into clothing if additional padding would be helpful. For rigidity there are sticks, tent poles, ice axes, stays from internal frame packs, ski poles. Some ensolite pads are rigid enough to make a padded splint when folded into place and secured around the arm or leg. Lightweight, commercial splints are available as additions to your backcountry first aid kit.

Splints can be secured in place with bandanas, strips of clothing, packs straps, belts, and pieces of rope. Useful items from your first aid kit for securing splints include tape and elastic wraps. Wide elastic wraps (6 inches) allow you to provide firm security with little loss of circulation. Large triangular bandages can be very helpful in the creation of slings and swathes.

Specific Fractures: Upper Body

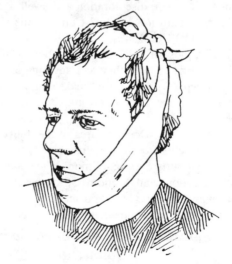

Figure 10–1
Stabilization method
for the jaw.

MANDIBLE (Jaw). Secure the jaw in place with a wide wrap that goes around the head. Be sure to provide for an adequate airway, and a way for the patient to quickly remove the wrap should they feel like vomiting (which they often do after a blow to the jaw).

CLAVICLE (Collarbone). You can break the thin collarbone with a direct blow or by falling on your arm or shoulder. The pain may be specific to the collarbone or general to the shoulder, and movement makes it worse. The

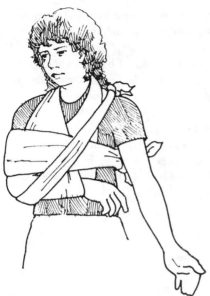

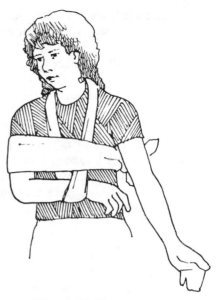

Figure 10–2a
Sling and swathes to stabilize a fractured
clavicle, lower arm, elbow, rib, etc.

Figure 10–2b
Sling and swathe to stabilize
a fractured humerus.

weight of the arm should be held firmly up in a sling. The sling should be
secured to the body with swathes to keep the shoulder immobile.

HUMERUS (Upper Arm). The upper arm bone can be broken with a direct
blow or a wrenching motion. Pain is usually specific to the damaged area, but
the patient may complain of shoulder pain if the fracture is high on the humerus.
Let the weight of the lower arm hang in a sling with the elbow free to hand down

Figure 10–3
Splint for the lower arm
or wrist.

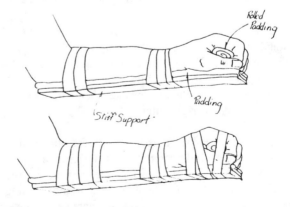

and pull a little traction of the injured upper arm. Wide wraps around the upper arm and chest secure the fracture to the rigid and well-padded chest wall.

RADIUS AND ULNA (Lower Arm). A fall or a direct blow to either bone of the lower arm may cause a fracture of one or both. Secure the lower arm to something well-padded and rigid, and hand the arm in a sling with swathes.

WRIST. If there is pain and swelling in the wrist, your suspicion of a fracture should be high. The complex structure of the wrist doesn't usually bend too far without breaking. Splint the lower arm being sure to incorporate the hand. Place a roll or wad of a soft material in the hand to keep in flexed into a position of function. Hang the arm in a sling with swathes.

HAND. Same as wrist.

FINGERS. The injured finger should be taped or wrapped securely to an adjacent finger after placing cotton or gauze between the fingers. Keep the fingers flexed in the normal position of function, not straight.

RIBS. Sling and swathe the arm on the injured side (see CHEST INJURIES).

Specific Fractures: Lower Body

PELVIS. In the backcountry, pelvic fractures are usually the result of falls from a height or high-speed skiing collisions. Pushing gently on the pelvis of the patient produces a marked pain response. Patients don't like to sit up or roll onto their side. There is the possibility of damage to internal organs and extensive internal bleeding. Pain can sometimes be reduced by wrapping the pelvis snugly. Splinting requires immobilization of the entire spinal column on a well-padded full backboard. Leg and body motion should be kept to a minimum. Sometimes a full backboard can be improvised from boards, straight sticks, or external pack frames lashed firmly together. Going for help is a healthy idea.

HIP. Fractures of the hip are not a common backcountry occurrence. Should it happen, the patient usually complains of pain very high on the femur (thigh) with their leg rolled outward from normal. Compare legs. With gentle traction, pull the broken leg into alignment with the other leg, pad well between the legs, and secure the two legs together. The patient will need to be carried out on a well-padded, rigid litter.

FEMUR (Thigh). This, your largest bone, takes a great deal of force to break. It usually takes a fall from a significant height or a very high-speed collision. There will be considerable pain in the region of the middle of the thigh. There can be considerable bleeding into the thigh. Prompt traction on the femur is required to 1) prevent an increase in the severity of the injury (an

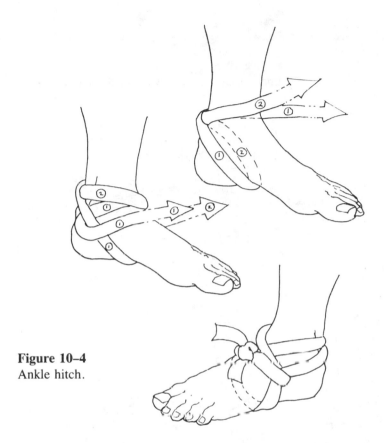

Figure 10–4
Ankle hitch.

unstable femur may even be pulled out through the skin by spasms of the muscles), 2) reduce bleeding into the thigh, and 3) reduce the amount of pain the patient is suffering. Unlike other fractures, the traction *cannot* be released after the tension is relieved in the muscle. The large thigh muscles may re-spasm violently.

Treatment of a fractured femur requires a device to maintain traction on the leg. Commercial products are available, but with creativity such a device can be improvised in the backcountry. While one rescuer maintains the manual traction, another gathers the material. A strip of something long and soft needs to be tied around the ankle on the injured leg with a loop at the sole of the foot. A shaft about one foot longer than the injured leg needs to be found. This can be a stick, a ski pole, a tent pole, a paddle. One end should be very well padded. Sometimes the shoe of the patient can be used for this pad. Secure the pad very well on the end of the shaft, and place the padded end gently in the groin of the patient. The patient may need a lot of reassurance. Secure the shaft in place near groin level with a wrap around the patient's upper thigh. A piece of rope, cord, or strong cloth is needed to make a trucker's hitch. Traction by the trucker's

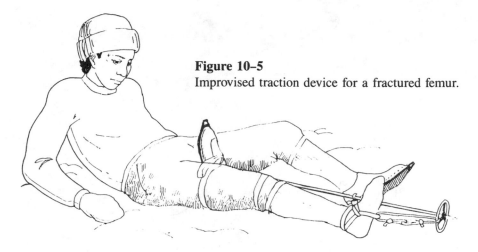

Figure 10–5
Improvised traction device for a fractured femur.

Figure 10–6
Trucker's Hitch.

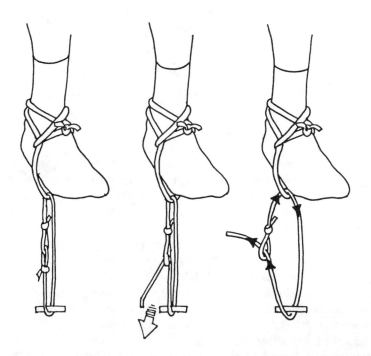

hitch is pulled from the loop at the sole of the foot and the end of the shaft until the traction of the device is equal or greater than the manual traction. The best judge of the amount of traction is the patient. They usually offer this judgment without your asking for it. When mechanical traction is secure, pad between the shaft and the leg, and use enough wraps of cloth or elastic bandages to secure the shaft firmly in place. If you find yourself alone with a victim suffering a fractured femur, you'll have to forego manual traction, gather the materials, and carefully apply mechanical traction when everything is in place. A rigid litter is usually required to get the patient out of the backcountry. The patient needs a hospital as soon as possible to prevent permanent of loss of function or loss of leg.

PATELLA (Kneecap). This is usually the result of a blow to the knee or falling on the knee. With a soft pad under the knee to keep the knee slightly flexed, the leg will need to be splinted. The knee often likes to be wrapped in a circular splint, one that wraps around the whole leg. Ensolite pads can work very well for this type of splint.

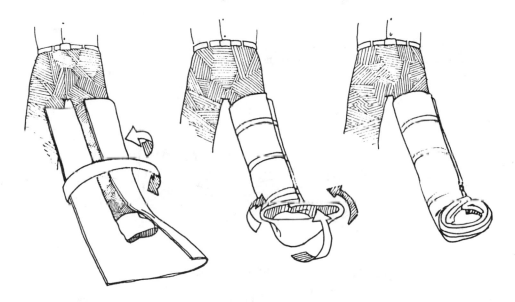

Figure 10–7
Improvised lower leg splint from an ensolite pad.

TIBIA AND FIBULA (Lower Leg). Lower leg fractures are most often the result of a high impact accident. The majority of backcountry evacuations for a musculoskeletal injury will be for a lower leg injury (knee, tibia, fibula, ankle). The splint should incorporate the knee and the ankle. Soft padding under the knee keeps the patient more comfortable. The rigidity should be concentrated under the leg where gravity's pull will be felt. An ensolite pad wrapped around the leg from above the knee and including the ankle, and tied firmly in place, will often suffice.

ANKLE. Any deformity, discoloration, or swelling that leaves an ankle unable to bear weight should be treated as a fracture. Remove the shoe and make a careful inspection. If needed, the foot should be placed in the position of function with gentle traction. Secure the ankle and foot in this position, or as close to it as possible.

FOOT. Same as ankle.

TOES. These little bones are usually damaged by violent stubs or something heavy being dropped on the toe and crushing the bone. Tape the toe to a healthy neighbor with cotton or gauze between the toes. Stiff-soled boots may enable the patient to walk out, or even continue the trip.

Figure 10–8
Traction-in-line to realign an angulated
fracture.

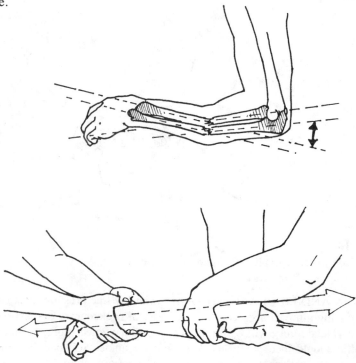

Complicated Fractures
Angulations

It is difficult to splint the unnaturally aligned bone. The patient suffers from pain and anguish over the deformity. Adequate circulation may be cut off by the angulation. For these reasons it is best to attempt to replace the bone in a natural alignment. The method is traction-in-line and reduction. Pulling slowly, steadily, and gently on the bone *along the line it is in* will relax the muscle, reduce the pain, and allow you to slowly move it gently into alignment. The sooner this attempt at reduction is made, the better. Do not continue if the patient complains of increasing pain. Do not continue if you have to use force to move it. Once aligned, splint as usual. If alignment cannot be achieved, splint it as best you can.

Open Fractures

When the bone shows, the situation is very serious. Surgical intervention is needed to save the extremity. After 6–8 hours, the possibility of loss of function or loss of limb goes up dramatically. Traction is not recommended since pulling the bone ends back under the skin increases the rate of infection. Rinsing the bone ends gently (not scrubbing), and covering them with a moist, sterile dressing is recommended. Splint as best you can and evacuate as soon as possible.

However, traction may be required if there is significant loss of life-giving circulation. An infected bone has a better chance of being saved than a bone that has died from lack of blood. Traction is also required on a fractured femur, even if the fracture is open. It is sometimes possible to pull the traction just enough to maintain stability without the ends of bone being drawn under the skin. Good luck!

Long-Term Fracture Care

Monitoring is the name of the game. Keep careful watch on the Circulation, Sensation, and Motion (CSM) of the injured arm or leg after the splint is in place. Swelling can cut off circulation, and require re-splinting. Time and the bouncing ride out on a litter can loosen a splint, and require re-splinting. It is important to give the patient the responsibility of letting you know if there are any changes in their condition.

The question of how fast to evacuate the fractured patient will depend on the situation and the severity of the injury. In all cases, a wise backcountry leader will have considered the possibilities beforehand. Ask yourself before leaving home: What can be done if such-and-such happens? What are our resources? Where is the closest aid, and how do we contact them? An extended carry is very strenuous even when you have a dozen people to switch off on the litter. And the extra gear may have to be carried as well.

Fractures that should be evacuated as soon as possible include 1) suspected spinal injuries, 2) pelvic injuries with suspected internal bleeding, 3) any open fracture, 4) a fractured femur or a high level of suspicion concerning one, and

5) any fracture with tremendous swelling and/or loss of circulation. Injuries involving the hip and knee are often associated with loss of function if left untreated for a long time.

The Barehanded Principles:
Fractures

1. *LAF (Look, Ask, and Feel) at the injury.*
   A. *Look for swelling, discoloration, asymmetry.*
   B. *ASK about pain, sensation, usability.*
   C. *FEEL for point tenderness, instability, pulse.*
2. *When in doubt, splint.*
3. *Splinting should include padding, something rigid, and should incorporate the joint above and below the injury unless the problem is isolated in a joint.*
4. *Angulations should be reduced with slow, steady, gentle traction-in-line.*
   A. *Use no force.*
   B. *Stop if pain increases.*
5. *Rinse and cover bone ends with a moist, sterile dressing, and splint as found unless circulation has been lost. Without Circulation, Sensation, and Motion (CSM), use gentle traction-in-line in an attempt to restore healthy blood flow.*
6. *Maintain manual traction on a fractured femur until a mechanical traction device can be applied.*
7. *Monitor the patient for changes in CSM, and keep track of their vital signs.*
8. *Evacuate.*

CHAPTER 11
DISLOCATIONS

Introduction

A period of melt-and-freeze temperatures had left the snowy surface hard, with just enough of a crust to hold weight a teasing moment before dropping the snowshoers through into softer underlying whiteness. For additional support, everyone was using two ski poles. It could have been frustrating, but the day's weather was pleasant, the group was congenial, and spirits were high. The walk up the ridge went quickly.

On the descent the trip went even quicker for Deborah. Her lighter weight kept her from crunching through on an especially dense crust in an opening on the steep forested hillside. She skied away from the group on her snowshoes. Planting a pole instinctively to brake herself, she slipped to the end of her arm's reach, and levered her right shoulder out of joint. Deborah plopped into a sitting position with a look of surprise that altered rapidly into one of intense pain. She sat huddled in the snow with her right arm cradled in her left. She was aware of what had happened to her. Her shoulder had been dislocated in the past.

It was a matter of moments before her friends had her lying back on an ensolite pad. Sitting in the snow beside her, a rescuer pulled gently on the arm on her injured side. The pull was in line with the way she held her arm. As the pressure on the pull was slowly increased, Deborah was encouraged to take deep breaths and relax her muscles.

With a soft and satisfying thump, the end of her upper arm bone rolled back into its socket. Her expression changed immediately to one of relief, and she released a long sigh.

Unzipping her parka about halfway, her arm was placed partially inside. The parka became a temporary sling. With the group sharing out her load, Deborah was able to snowshoe to the van, about two miles distant. A short visit to the hospital revealed nothing extraordinary in her shoulder. She went home with soreness but no serious damage.

Any joint of the body can come out of joint. The mechanism of injury can be indirect (the stuck ski pole levers out a shoulder, the high brace of the kayaker pries out a shoulder) or direct (a fall on a shoulder knocks it out). If the bones stay locked out of normal alignment, the injury is a dislocation (a dis-lock-ation). Direct mechanisms tend to cause more damage to the joint because of the forces involved.

Assessment

As with any musculoskeletal injury, have a good LAF at the patient (See FRACTURES). Look for deformity, and asymmetry. A dislocated joint just doesn't look like the patient's normally aligned joints. Look for guarding. Patients tend to protect injured joints. Ask about pain. Dislocations are typically very painful. Ask about ability to move. A dislocation prevents the normal range of motion in the joint. Feel for a pain response and deformity. Sometimes a rescuer's hand will "see" things that eyes have missed.

Look, Ask, and Feel (LAF) for adequate circulation beyond the dislocation. The skin should look healthy in color. The patient should not complain of numbness or tingling. There should be a pulse beyond the dislocation. Loss of circulation is the major serious complication with a dislocation, and a cause for determined action.

Treatment

Work quickly but calmly. The sooner an attempt to relocate, or reduce the angle of dislocation, is made, the easier it will be for you and the patient. She will feel better, and her joint will receive an adequate blood supply, if the relocation is successful. You need to get the patient to relax as much as possible. Ask her to take deep breaths, and let all the tension go from the painful area. Have her lie down. Lightly touch the dislocation, reminding the patient where to concentrate her attempt to relax.

Be assured, if you work steadily and gently, the patient's condition will be made better, not worse. Fractures, blood vessel damage, and nerve impairment often associated with dislocations will be improved by a non-forceful relocation. And the evacuation will be easier and safer for everyone involved.

Place yourself comfortably in a position allowing you to pull gentle traction-in-line. Taking a firm grip on the arm (or leg), lean your body weight slowly back, pulling *in line* with the way the patient is holding her extremity. Keeping your arms straight will allow you to relax more than trying to pull with the strength of your arms only. DO NOT USE FORCE. STOP IF PAIN IN-CREASES.

If the dislocation does not relocate after you've pulled traction-in-line for a minute, gently move the extremity away from the patient's body. Maintain traction during the movement. What you're trying to do is manually relax the muscular spasms, and move the bones toward a normal alignment. You can move the bones toward a more normal alignment as long as the patient does not complain of increasing pain, and you're not forcing movement. The muscles, tendons, and ligaments "want" to be back where they belong. You're encouraging them to move back. The patient will tell you when relocation has occurred. Most relocated dislocations need to be immobilized (See SPLINTING) until a physician can examine the injury.

Occasionally a dislocation will be severe enough to prevent relocation. You will have to splint the extremity in the position the patient is holding it. Make the splint as comfortable as possible. Evacuate the patient as soon as you can.

Specific Dislocations: Upper Body

MANDIBLE (Jaw). After wrapping something soft and protective around your thumbs, reach gently into the patient's mouth, gripping the back molars. Pull down and forward until relocation occurs.

CERVICAL SPINE (Neck). Any deformity or loss of motion in the neck qualifies the patient for treatment as a spinal cord injury (See SPINAL CORD INJURY MANAGEMENT).

SHOULDER. With the patient lying down, pull gentle traction-in-line on the arm. The pressure of the traction may cause the patient to slide across the ground, and require a second rescuer to wrap a shirt or parka around the chest of the patient in order to apply traction in the opposite direction. Moving toward normal alignment mimics the motion the arm of the patient would go through if she were a student raising her hand to answer a question in class. Once relocated, immobilize the shoulder with the arm in a sling, if possible. Secure the sling with swathes or a wide elastic wrap.

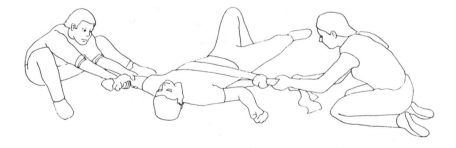

Figure 11–1
A traction method for reduction of a dislocated shoulder.

In the absence of a second rescuer, or with difficult relocations, the patient can be placed prone across a rock or log with the arm on the injured side hanging down with about 15 pounds of weight tied to the hand. It may be a long wait, but the muscles will usually fatigue in time, allowing the shoulder to relocate.

It is not a healthy idea for you to place one of your feet in the patient's armpit, and pull aggressively on the arm. The abundant blood vessels and nerves of the armpit can easily be damaged.

ELBOW. Traction-in-line is easiest applied by two rescuers, one holding above the elbow, and the other holding below, with the injured arm flexed. An elbow can be dislocated to the inside or outside, and may require side pressure to the joint as well as traction-in-line. Once relocated, sling and swathe the injured arm.

WRIST. Dislocated wrists are usually fractured. They should be placed in normal alignment, and splinted.

FINGERS. Keeping the finger partially flexed, pull on the end while actually pushing the dislocated joint back into place. This is safe, and easier than just pulling. Pad between the injured finger and a healthy neighbor, and tape the two fingers together.

Dislocations of the base of the fingers, where they join the hand, are difficult to relocate, and often require surgery. Treatment may be limited to splinting the hand, and evacuating the patient.

Specific Dislocations: Lower Body

HIP. This relocation requires two rescuers, and still may prove impossible. Large muscle masses are involved. With the patient on her back, one rescuer straddles her body and lifts the leg on the injured side at the knee to flexion of 90 degrees. The other rescuer pushes down firmly on the patient's pelvis. If reduction occurs, pad between the patient's legs, and tie the legs together. The evacuation will be a carry-out instead of a walk-out.

KNEE. With gentle traction, move the leg to a normal alignment. Splint the injured leg securely, and carry the patient out.

PATELLA (Kneecap). Apply gentle traction in order to straighten out the injured leg. Sometime the kneecap will pop back into place when the leg is straightened. If not, push it back into place. This may require some gentle force, but the patella is not a normal joint, and force is safely applied here. With a circular splint from groin to ankle, the patient may be comfortable enough to hobble out using an improvised crutch.

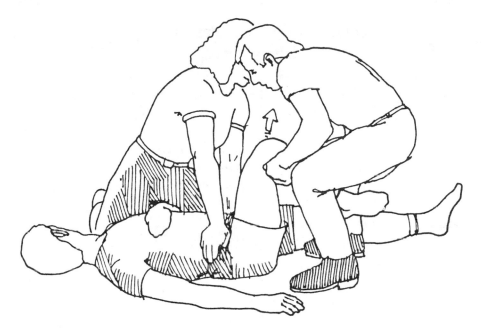

Figure 11-2
Method for attempting reduction of a dislocated hip.

ANKLE. Dislocated ankles are usually very unstable and easily realigned with traction. Ankles are also highly susceptible to de-circulation, and every effort should be made to return the joint to normal alignment. Gentle traction can be applied at the foot and heel. A second rescuer pulling on the lower leg would be useful, but the weight of the patient is usually enough counterpressure to allow the relocation without a second rescuer. The patient will require carrying.

TOES. Same as fingers.

Long-Term Dislocation Care
Regular monitoring is required to ensure your patient maintains adequate circulation to the injured area. Check often for a pulse beyond the injured joint, and normal skin color and sensations beyond the joint. Give the patient the responsibility of notifying you of changes in their condition.

Most dislocations should be evacuated for careful medical examination even if they relocate easily. There is always the chance of underlying damage that doesn't show up right away, especially with first time dislocations. Exceptions would include fingers and toes, and chronic dislocations (repeat offenders) that the patient is able to use with reasonable comfort after the relocation.

The Barehanded Principles:
Dislocations

1. *LAF (Look, Ask, and Feel) at the injury.*
   A. *Look for deformity and asymmetry.*
   B. *Ask about pain and loss of ability to move.*
   C. *Feel for tenderness and deformity.*
2. *Encourage the patient to relax.*
3. *Place the patient comfortably on the ground.*
4. *Pull gentle traction-in-line on the dislocated bones.*
5. *Under traction, move the bones toward normal alignment.*
6. *Do not use force.*
7. *Stop if pain increases.*
8. *Whether you achieve relocation or not, splint the injured joint.*
9. *Monitor the patient for changes indicating loss of circulation.*
10. *Evacuate.*

CHAPTER 12
ENVIRONMENTAL EMERGENCIES

Introduction

The ENVIRONMENTAL EMERGENCIES are medical conditions that are induced when the human body is stressed, by environmental factors, beyond its normal limitations. As a result, the thermoregulatory system can no longer maintain a proper core temperature and life threatening situations may ensue.

The cornerstone of understanding these emergencies is an appreciation of the THERMOREGULATORY SYSTEM of the human body, its limitations, and what happens when those limitations are exceeded.

As a species, we are warm-blooded animals, which means that we expend a great deal of energy simply maintaining a constant core temperature. The ability to maintain a consistent core temperature allows us to function in a variety of environmental conditions. This constant core temperature is maintained by our "thermoregulatory system". If our core temperature begins to rise or fall, protective mechanisms react to return our temperature to normal.

The thermoregulatory center is located at the base of the brain in the brainstem. Although it constantly monitors the temperature of the blood as an indicator of our core temperature, the brainstem itself does not have the ability to adjust the core temperature. The affector organs that adjust the core temperature are the skin and circulatory system.

With many important functions, the skin is the largest organ of the human body. One of its most important functions is the maintenance of a constant core temperature. Under the direction of the brain, the skin has the ability to lose excess heat if our core temperature begins to rise or to conserve heat if our core temperature begins to fall.

Of these two extremes, heat and cold, the human body is better adapted at dealing with the heat. Until relatively recent history, humans have resided primarily in the tropical and subtropical locales, where it was easiest to survive and thrive. Because we evolved in a hot, tropical environment it was essential that we develop a very efficient cooling system. With few exceptions, ours is one of the most effective and unique cooling systems for any animal species.

Also, as a result of evolving in a hot climate, a method to conserve heat was not a necessary development. Having less effective mechanisms for heat conservation, we are more predisposed to cold injury than heat injury.

In order to maintain a constant core temperature, the thermoregulatory center in the brainstem has to balance heat production against heat loss.

Heat Production

BASAL METABOLIC RATE: The basal metabolic rate (BMR) is the constant rate at which the human body consumes energy to drive chemical reactions and produce heat to maintain life at a constant core temperature. It is the BMR that maintains us at 98.6F.

NUTRITION and HYDRATION: Food and water are the fuels that are burned to maintain the BMR.

EXERCISE: The activity of using muscles consumes energy and produces heat faster than normal, thus increasing the core temperature and requiring cooling mechanisms to be employed.

Heat Loss

CONDUCTION: Heat is lost from a warmer object to a colder object via conduction. The extreme form of conductive heat loss is a warm body placed in cold water. This can increase the rate of heat loss 20–30 times.

CONVECTION: Heat is lost directly into the air. The extreme form of convective heat loss is windchill. In this case the warm body has heated the air surrounding it, but that warm air is replaced by cold air blowing around it. This

Figure 12–1
Balancing heat production against heat loss.

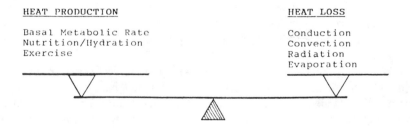

HEAT PRODUCTION   HEAT LOSS

Basal Metabolic Rate   Conduction
Nutrition/Hydration   Convection
Exercise   Radiation
                                                   Evaporation

THERMOREGULATORY CENTER

increases the rate at which the warm body loses heat. Windchill can increase heat loss 5–10 times.

EVAPORATION: As water evaporates it requires energy to convert from a liquid to a gas, which can increase the rate of heat loss 20–30 times. This is our most important cooling mechanisms since it accounts for greater than 90% of our cooling efficiency.

RADIATION: Heat is given off by a warm object as infrared energy. Radiational cooling can increase heat loss several times.

With these few principles in mind let's look at how heat and cold can tax the resources of the human body. Decreasing our ability to perform and possibly producing life-threatening emergencies.

CHAPTER 13
HEAT INJURY AND ILLNESS

The blueberries were plentiful and ripe under the late July sun. John, Jan, and David were looking forward to a hike in the mountains to this favorite spot.

Saturday finally arrived and they managed to get off to an early start. The hike they were planning was approximately 3 miles long with a gain of elevation of 3500 feet. It would take them to an exposed ridged covered with blueberry bushes. Since they had been on this trail before, they knew that there would not be any water, so they each carried a quart of water. The day was spectacular—clear, warm, and sunny with a gentle breeze higher up.

Reaching their destination by noontime, each was soaked with sweat from the exertion of the climb. They sat like bears among the blueberries and enjoyed a drink of cool water and the taste of the ripe fruit. For several hours they simply nibbled and collected blueberries, reveling in the summer warmth and the surrounding beauty.

Towards midafternoon David started complaining of thirst and decided it was time to descend in search of water. Normally it would have taken them about an hour to cover the 3 miles, but on this day it took several hours and required an unusual amount of effort and exertion for all three.

Once down, they simply sat next to the car exhausted. Both John and Jan felt slightly nauseous and light-headed. David, on the other hand, was beginning to act strange, slightly disoriented and very argumentative. He stated firmly that he was hot, tired, and very thirsty. With that, they loaded up the car and headed out.

As they drove towards home David became more and more disoriented and combative. His skin was red, hot, and dry. He began to rant and appeared to be hallucinating. Appropriately, his companions decided to drive him to the local hospital emergency room where he was admitted to the intensive care unit.

This incident involves all three of the heat-related emergencies: dehydration, heat exhaustion, and heat stroke.

Dehydration

We assume that our thirst mechanism will protect us from dehydration, that if we become dehydrated it will tell us by causing intense thirst that will not diminish until we are properly hydrated. But this isn't always the case. It is possible to lose fluid so quickly that the normal thirst mechanism is overwhelmed or overridden.

The sources of fluid loss are respiration, perspiration, urination, and defecation. The rate of loss from each of these will vary according to activity levels, air temperature, humidity, and altitude.

RESPIRATION: With normal daily activities we lose approximately 1–2 liters of water via evaporation from the lungs. As we breathe, the air that we inhale is "conditioned"—it is warmed to 98.6 F and humidified to 100% humidity. This warm, moist air is then exhaled and the cycle started over again. The combination of extreme cold temperatures and altitude can dramatically increase the rate of water loss through the lungs, up to 1 cup per hour or 6 liters in 24 hours.

PERSPIRATION: With normal daily activities we do not sweat very hard so the loss is minimal, about 1–2 liters per day. But with exertion in hot, dry weather, this can become extreme. During heavy exertion, we can lose 1–2 liters of water per hour which can easily amount to 8–10 liters of fluid while exercising.

URINATION: 1–2 liters of fluid are lost daily via urination to clear waste products from the blood. The amount of urine produced will increase with overhydration and decrease with dehydration.

DEFECATION: The average daily loss of fluid through defecation is approximately 0.1 liter. This can increase dramatically with diarrhea to as much as 25 liters in a 24-hour period.

Through the activities of daily living, the average day's loss of fluid is 4 liters, which is generally replaced by the fluid we drink and the food we eat. But, the amount of fluid required can be significantly increased by exercise, sweating, diarrhea, temperature, or altitude. The most common cause of increased fluid loss is exercise and sweating. Sweating alone can increase fluid requirements to 8–16 liters per day or 2–4 gallons of replacement fluid.

John, Jan, and David thought they were prepared with their 1 quart of water each. They did not appreciate the amount of fluid that they would lose from sweating or the effects that dehydration would have on them. One quart simply was not enough fluid to replace the 3–4 liters each had lost hiking and sitting in the hot summer sun. By mid-afternoon, when David began to complain, they were already dehydrated and suffering the consequences.

Figure 13-1
Comparing the water normally
taken in during a day outdoors to
the water the body loses.

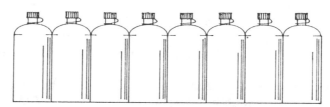

The effects of dehydration are, decreased physical ability, fatigue, and impairment of judgment and thinking ability. These factors increased the difficulty of the hike out and could have led to a physical mishap or becoming lost.

Once down to the trailhead, though, they each displayed other heat-related injuries besides dehydration, which their dehydration contributed to. Jan and John appeared heat exhausted and David's illness progressed to heat stroke.

Heat Injury

In the process of hiking uphill, Jan, John, and David all began to overheat from the exertion. As our body core temperature begins to rise, our thermoregulatory system engages the cooling mechanisms. The excess heat building up from muscle activity is absorbed by the blood. As the thermoregulatory center in the brainstem detects the increase in blood temperature, the brain causes the peripheral circulation, the vasculature of the skin, to dilate, or open up. This dilation of peripheral vasculature increases the blood flow to the skin where the blood can be cooled. At the same time, to further increase the rate of heat loss from the skin, the brain stimulates the sweat glands to produce sweat. The evaporation of sweat from the skin increases the rate of cooling many times.

Sweat consists primarily of water and some electrolytes, specifically sodium and chloride ions. As long as we can sweat and the sweat can evaporate, we can continue to cool ourselves efficiently. But, if for some reason, either the sweating mechanism begins to fail or the sweat cannot evaporate, then the cooling mechanism will fail.

On hot, very humid days our cooling mechanism is extremely inefficient and it becomes relatively easy to overheat because the sweat cannot evaporate. The evaporation of sweat from the skin accounts for 90% of our cooling ability. Additionally, our ability to sweat diminishes as we become dehydrated.

Heat Exhaustion

Jan and John both experienced heat exhaustion, a condition caused by water and electrolyte loss. The primary cause of symptoms appears to be related to the amount of sodium and chloride ions rather than the amount of water lost.

Heat exhaustion is not a life-threatening illness. As with Jan and John, symptoms include fatigue, exhaustion, nausea, lightheadedness, and possibly heat cramps. Heat exhaustion usually comes on several hours after exertion and dehydration. The individual may have even replaced the lost fluids but not the electrolytes.

With about twelve hours of rest, heat exhaustion is self-correcting. However, this condition can be treated rapidly with an electrolyte solution consisting of one teaspoon of table salt (sodium chloride) dissolved in a quart of water, which should be slowly sipped over a period of 15 minutes. The salt water mixture can be administered several more times, and complete recovery should occur within 1 hour.

Salt tablets are too concentrated, and should be avoided. They draw water into the stomach to dilute the salt, while the sufferer needs the water out in the circulatory system where it is used to help maintain a normal core temperature.

The cramps sometimes associated with heat exhaustion are painful but not damaging to the patient unless the cramps are ignored and the sufferer pushes on. As with any cramp, they can be massaged away. Drinking the salty water and resting should keep them from reappearing.

Prevention

Heat exhaustion can be avoided by consuming enough water to replace the fluids lost, and eating salty foods or drinking an electrolyte solution. Drink because you know you should, not because you feel thirst. Keep yourself and your group at a pace that allows your body to adapt to the heat. If you feel the symptoms of exhaustion coming on, you're going too fast. It is especially important to pace yourself early in the hot, humid season. Your thermoregulatory system will become more efficient as it gets used to summer. Take a break during the hottest part of the day, the middle afternoon hours. Wear cotton clothing that lets air pass through and sweat evaporate. And wear a brimmed hat or cap to shade your heat conscious head.

Heat Stroke

Heat stroke, on the other hand, is a life-threatening emergency. Without proper care heat stroke victims will most likely die. David displayed the classic signs and symptoms of heat stroke. David's situation is more severe than his companions because he became so dehydrated that he was unable to produce sweat and, consequently, lost his ability to cool off.

Once our cooling mechanism fails, our core temperature begins to rise rapidly. Death can occur in as little as 30 minutes. With the rising core temperature, the brain, which can only exist in a very narrow temperature range, begins to fail. In an effort to cool the blood and lower the core temperature, the brain will dilate all the blood vessels in the skin. As a result, the skin becomes RED, HOT, and may be DRY.

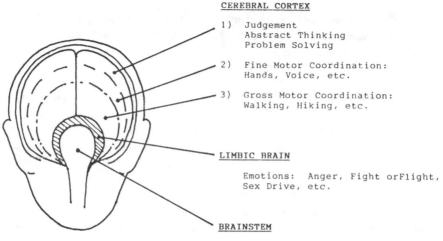

CEREBRAL CORTEX

1) Judgement
   Abstract Thinking
   Problem Solving

2) Fine Motor Coordination:
   Hands, Voice, etc.

3) Gross Motor Coordination:
   Walking, Hiking, etc.

LIMBIC BRAIN

Emotions: Anger, Fight orFlight,
Sex Drive, etc.

BRAINSTEM

Cardiovascular Center
Respiratory Center
Thermoregulation Center
Reticular Activating Center

Figure 13–2
Evolution has added layer after
layer of increasing mental prowess
onto our brains.

As the brain overheats, the individual may become disoriented, combative, argumentative, and may hallucinate wildly. David exhibited all of these symptoms and was appropriately taken to the local emergency room. But, heat stroke treatment should be begun immediately.

The primary goal of therapy is to cool the victim as rapidly as possible. Since the sweating mechanism has failed, we have to sweat for them. The simplest and most efficient method is to soak the victim with water, fanning them to increase the rate of evaporation, and massaging their extremities to encourage the return of cool blood to the core. With a limited supply of water, cooling the head becomes the top priority. All heat stroke victims must be transported to the hospital as quickly as possible, continuing the cooling process during evacuation.

Heat stroke victims are dehydrated and require rehydration. Unfortunately, getting them to drink may be impossible. With their impaired mental condition, it is inappropriate to force fluids on them. If they refuse to drink, continue cooling them externally.

Prevention

Heat stroke, like all the heat related injuries, is preventable. The same prevention methods that work for dehydration and exhaustion, will work for heat stroke. The guiding principles is to stay well hydrated. Do not rely upon your thirst mechanism to tell you when and how much you need to drink. Under conditions of exertion, it is probably impossible to drink too much water. Four quarts per day is certainly a reasonable minimum goal.

The Barehanded Principles:
Heat Injury

1. *Stay well hydrated and munch salty snacks.*
2. *Rest often out of the heat.*
3. *Wear clothing that allows evaporation, and a brimmed hat or cap.*
4. *Give heat exhausted patients lots of water with a teaspoon of salt per quart. And let them rest.*
5. *Cool heat stroke victims as rapidly as possible pouring on water, fanning, and massaging the extremities. And evacuate them.*

CHAPTER 14
COLD INJURIES

As was mentioned earlier, we are, as a species, better adapted to dealing with heat than with cold because we evolved in the tropical and subtropical environs with minimal exposure to cold conditions. As a result, our protective mechanisms for dealing with heat loss situations are not as efficient.

The same thermoregulatory center in the brain that monitors the blood/core temperature for excessive heat gain also gauges the rate of heat loss. When we begin to lose heat faster than we are producing it, and our core temperature begins to fall below normal, the brain will activate protective mechanisms designed to prevent any further heat loss. If the temperature continues to fall, the brain will employ further measures in an attempt to reheat the body.

It snowed last night in the higher elevations, creating a spectacular view of lightly dusted mountaintops. A magnificent sight greeted Peter and Alphonso as they crawled out of their sleeping bags into the crisp morning air.

Anxious to get started, they had a quick breakfast of hot chocolate and bagels, packed up their gear, and were off to chase the snow line several thousand feet above them.

Both Peter and Alphonso had some experience in hiking and camping, but little experience in winter camping. What they lacked in experience they made up for in enthusiasm. Before long, they were stripped down to their T-shirts in an effort to stay cool while rushing uphill to reach the summit. An occasional stop to snack on cheese and bread and sip water served to add fuel to their fire and replace some of the fluid lost to sweat. Several hours later they found themselves at the snowline, with a gentle cool breeze and a slightly overcast sky.

Now hiking in about 6 inches of snow, they estimated that they would summit by noon. Their pace slowed as the temperature dropped and the breeze changed to a cold wind. Alphonso was the first to suggest that they stop and put on some warmer clothing. As Alphonso put on a pile top and a wind breaker, Peter explained that he was not cold and the additional clothing would only cause him to start sweating again.

The hour to the summit turned into several. Finally, at about 2 in the afternoon, Peter and Alphonso reached the top in a fog. They sat there on the snow-covered rocks sipping their last bit of water hoping to catch a glimpse of the valleys below.

After 30 minutes Alphonso suggested that they head down in order to make their car before nightfall. Peter, slowly getting up, complained that his feet were cold and started down, leaving his pack behind. Alphonso stopped him and had to assist him with putting his pack on.

On the way down Peter became very quiet. Occasionally stumbling at first, his walk slowly turned into a constant stagger. His speech became slurred and he no longer made sense. He seemed unaware of the cold, and began falling into the snow with regularity. Alphonso noticed that each time he helped Peter out of the snow and back to his feet Peter made little or no effort to brush the snow from his clothing.

By nightfall they had reached their previous campsite. Peter was useless. Alphonso sat him under a tree and proceeded to set up their tent. With great effort he managed to get Peter into the tent and into a sleeping bag. Tired and hungry, Alphonso crawled into his bag for a fitful night's sleep.

Come morning, Alphonso was unable to arouse Peter, and eventually decided his best course of action was to leave Peter in his sleeping bag and go for help.

Sixteen hours later the rescue team arrived to find an apparently lifeless Peter. However, recognizing severe hypothermia, they treated Peter appropriately and evacuated him to the hospital. The evacuation took 12 hours.

At the hospital Peter was treated for severe hypothermia and frostbite. He was released from the hospital 35 days after admission, minus a few toes.

Hypothermia

Hypothermia is a condition where the body has continued to lose heat faster than it was producing heat long enough to depress the core temperature. As a result the brain and the body both begin to fail.

The most susceptable organ in the human body to a lowered core temperature is the brain which is designed to function optimally at 98.6 degrees. If the temperature is elevated above or lowered below this ideal temperature, the brain will malfunction. In the case of hypothermia, the thought processes will become impaired.

Evolution has added layer after layer of increasing mental prowess onto our brains, with the newest and most advanced layer being the outermost layer. The original primitive brain, in the center, is the brainstem. Housed in the brainstem are all of the functions required to live from second to second and minute to minute—the respiratory center which sets our respiratory rate; the cardiovascular center which sets our heart rate; the thermoregulatory center that sets our core temperature; and the reticular activating center that establishes our level of consciousness.

Surrounding the brainstem is the limbic brain, also a primitive part of the brain, which houses the functions that allow us to survive from month-to-month, year-to-year, and to survive as a species. The centers for emotions, anger, posturing, rudimentary defenses of fight or flight, and sex drive that allows the species to propagate and continue are found in the limbic brain.

Encasing the limbic brain is the newest addition to the brain, the cerebral cortex. This layer controls gross motor functions like the ability to walk and run; fine motor functions such as the ability to build and use tools; our hands and voice, areas dedicated to problem-solving, abstract thinking and judgement, and areas alert to the awareness of dangers and the environment.

As the brain becomes impaired by cold various functions begin to fail, starting with the outermost layer and progressing inward. The first things to go are our awareness of danger and the environment, problem-solving, and judgement, and it is these cognitive functions that protect us from danger and prevent us from getting injured or lost in the woods.

The increasing impairment of the brain, as the core temperature falls below normal is from the newest and most complex functions of the brain to the oldest most rudimentary processes of life.

98.6F—Intact mental and physical functions.

96F —Confusion.
        Apathy.
        SHIVERING begins as a fine uncontrollable motor tremor.
        Loss of problem-solving ability.
        Decreased self-awareness and self protection.
        Skin becomes pale and cool.

94F —Occasional stumbling.
        SHIVERING continues and becomes an obvious shaking tremor.
        Little or no effort made to protect self.
        Little or no recognition of the present situation.

92F —Difficulty walking/frequent stumbling.
        SHIVERING increases in intensity.
        No effort made to protect self.
        Speech becomes thick.
        Hallucinations may occur.
        Skin appears dusky gray and cold.

90F —Walking impossible.
   SHIVERING is convulsive, coming it waves.
   Speech is very thick and difficult to understand.

86F —All SHIVERING activity has ceased.
   Pulse and respirations appear to be absent ("METABOLIC ICEBOX").
   Skin is now cyanotic (blue).

When the brain first sensed that the body was losing heat faster than the body was producing it, it stimulated the primary defense mechanism against further heat loss—VASOCONSTRICTION of the peripheral circulation.

This vasoconstriction of the peripheral circulation occurs in the skin, the affector organ of the thermoregulatory system. The minute blood vessels near the surface of the skin contract, preventing blood from reaching the surface of the skin where it will lose heat into the surrounding environment. The lack of blood causes the skin to become pale and cool.

If the core temperature continues to fall, the brain will stimulate the muscles to contract and relax or "shiver", a form of involuntary exercise designed to consume energy and produce heat without requiring work. As the core temperature continues to fall, the brain will increase the intensity of shivering in an effort to rewarm itself.

As long as victims are actively trying to rewarm themselves, they will shiver. For simplicity, shivering victims can be considered mildly hypothermic. As the temperature continues to drop the shivering mechanism will not be able to produce enough heat to keep up with the heat loss, or the muscles will run out of fuel to burn to maintain the shivering. How long the defenses can hold up against the cold depends upon the rate of heat loss. When shivering stops, patients have lost the ability to rewarm themselves. Without help, they will probably die. They can be considered severely hypothermic.

Treatment of Hypothermia

1. For the mildly hypothermic victim almost anything that helps them create and maintain heat will help: fluid replacement, food (especially simple carbohydrates), exercise, external heat sources (ie. fire). But remember TO STAY WARM YOU MUST STAY DRY. Change their wet clothing to dry. If you crawl into a sleeping bag with a mildly hypothermic person, wear lightweight clothing so your normothermic sweat doesn't dampen their hypothermic body.

2. If your victim is severely hypothermic, no longer actively generating heat, seek out or create a stable environment. This can be a tent, snow cave, bivouac shelter, or cabin. Just as it is impossible to treat a burn victim in a burning building, it is impossible to treat a cold injury in a freezer.

3. Handle the patient gently. Rough physical movement can cause their cold heart to stop. Strip the damp clothing off. If the victim remains wet or damp, they cannot be rewarmed.

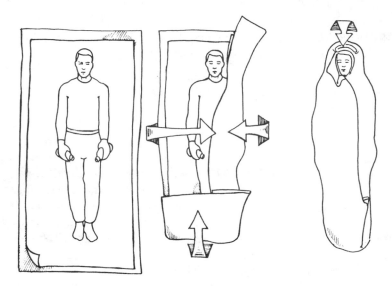

Figure 14–1
Hypothermia wrap.

4. Surround them with a HYPOTHERMIA WRAP.
   A. First step: Insulate them from the cold ground with an ensolite pad and surround them with multiple layers of insulation. What you insulate them with does not matter as long as it is dry.
   B. Second step: If possible, place warm water bottles or heat packs in their hands and/or at neck, armpits and groin.
   C. Third step: Prevent convectional and radiational heat loss by wrapping them in anything windproof and waterproof.
   D. Pay attention to details. It is absolutely essential that the victim be completely surrounded by all layers. Protect the head where heat loss can be extreme. The only thing exposed to the environment should be their face.

5. If they are conscious and able to swallow without fear of aspiration, give them a sickly sweet liquid to sip. The shivering process consumes large amounts of energy. Muscles need sugar to shiver, and we need to replace the sugar being used up. If we do not keep adding logs to the fire, the fire will go out and the person will die. The hypothermia victim may not be able to digest solids but will be able to absorb liquids. One of the easiest and most efficient products to use is Jello. In a metal cup warm a cup of water and dissolve the Jello, so that you end up with a sickly sweet drink.

6. If the victim is unconscious or goes unconscious, do not attempt to give them anything by mouth. Hypothermia wrap them and seek help for evacuation.

Hypothermia is the leading cause of backcountry emergencies, injuries, and searches. The first and most important effect of hypothermia is that it impairs the level of judgement and blunts our natural protective instincts. As a result we become lost, unaware of the environment and changing weather patterns, and take chances. To risk hypothermia is to risk injury in an unforgiving environment where help is not immediately available.

Prevention of Hypothermia

Understand hypothermia and our susceptability to it.

Don't go out unprepared. Carry extra warm clothing, a warm hat and mittens. Wear the clothing in layers, taking off the outer layer before warming up and sweating, and adding them back on before cooling off.

Be aware of changing weather patterns. Put on your rain gear before it starts to rain.

Be aware of each other. Hypothermia occurs with little or no warning to the victim.

Eat often. You need fuel to burn to stay warm.

Drink often. Staying well hydrated is just as important as staying well fed.

Know your limitations. Realize that we are not well adapted to the cold, and that we have to rely upon extra equipment and resources to survive.

Frostbite

Frostbite is localized tissue damage caused by the cold. It creates a spectrum of injuries depending on how cold the tissue becomes. Ranging from little or no damage to extensive damage resulting in tissue loss, this spectrum of injuries can be classified in two basic categories: superficial frostbite or deep frostbite.

Before considering these two types of frostbite, it is worth exploring why humans appear to be more susceptable to frostbite than other animals.

Actually the answer is quite simple, a question of priorities between physical abilities or mental prowess. As a finger begins to cool off, for example, because of a hole in a mitten, it will send signals to the brain relaying its predicament. In essence, it is asking the brain to dilate the blood vessels leading to it which would then increase the blood flow and bring warm blood out to it. The brain now has to make a choice. The brain could increase the circulation to the finger. But, if the brain sends warm blood out to the tip of that cold finger, in an effort to rewarm it, the blood returning from that finger will be cold. Cold blood creates the risk of hypothermia, and hypothermia impairs the brain. To impair the brain is to risk injury or worse to the entire self.

The brain will not risk hypothermia to save the finger. In fact, it will constrict the blood vessels going out to the cold finger to further reduce the possibility of hypothermia, increasing the risk and severity of frostbite to the finger.

The initial stage of frostbite is SUPERFICIAL FROSTBITE. This occurs when the tissues are damaged by the cold but do not freeze solid like a block of ice. Problems occur when the water within the cells expands as it begins to freeze causing the cells to rupture.

The signs and symptoms of superficial frostbite are pale skin and numbness, both due to decreased circulation to the area. Even though the area is pale and numb, it is still soft and pliable to the touch. Superficial frostbite can be field-treated.

Treatment consists of skin-to-skin rewarming. The cold area should be in contact with warm skin. For example, a cold finger can be cradled in a warm armpit, or cold feet placed against the warm belly of your backcountry partner.

Occasionally when superficial frostbite is rewarmed, a large fluid-filled blister, called a BLEB, forms. If this occurs, do not pop the blister. Leave it intact. Insulate the area well with dry material to prevent refreezing and evacuate.

If frostbite is not treated in the superficial stage, it can progress to DEEP FROSTBITE. Deep frostbite can be recognized because the affected area is frozen solid. This type of severe frostbite should not be field rewarmed. The thawing of deep frostbite is extremely painful and must be monitored in a definitive care facility. Instead the frostbitten section should be insulated well to prevent any further freezing or rewarming and the victim evacuated.

Prevention

As with hypothermia, frostbite is preventable. Unlike other mammals, we are not covered with a warm fur coat. Instead we have to carry it with us. The first rule in prevention of frostbite is to have the proper clothing for the environment we are going into and know how to use it. Ideal clothing will insulate well even when wet. It will not be constrictive, especially in the feet where humans are most susceptible to cold damage. There should be extra clothing available if we do get wet.

The second rule is to pay attention to your body. As soon as a cold or numb area is seen or felt, rewarm it to prevent superficial frostbite from becoming severe deep frostbite.

The Barehanded Principles:
Cold Injury

1. STAY WELL HYDRATED: Dehydration increases the risk of all the environmental emergencies, as well as inducing fatigue and impairing mental abilities.

2. HYPOTHERMIA IS THE LEADING CAUSE OF BACKCOUNTRY ACCIDENTS:
   A. Stay dry and carry raingear.
   B. Eat often and drink water often.
   C. Carry extra warm clothing.

    D. *Watch the weather.*

    E. *KNOW YOUR LIMITATIONS.*

3. *TO TREAT HYPOTHERMIA:*

    A. *Get into a stable environment.*

    B. *DRY OFF THE VICTIM.*

    C. *HYPOTHERMIA WRAP the victim.*

    D. *If conscious feed the victim a sickly sweet liquid.*

    E. *If unconscious, evacuate GENTLY as soon as possible.*

4. *TO PREVENT FROSTBITE:*

    A. *Stay well hydrated.*

    B. *Use proper clothing for the conditions.*

    C. *Rewarm cold areas early with passive skin-to-skin contact.*

5. *IF DEEP FROSTBITE OCCURS:*

    A. *Do not attempt to field rewarm.*

    B. *Dry off and reinsulate the area to prevent further injury.*

    C. *Evacuate.*

CHAPTER 15
LIGHTNING

Introduction

It was a popular campsite, proven safe by years of unremarkable usage. The July storm, rolling in around 1:30 AM, brought heavy rain and booming claps of thunder. After a particularly close lightning strike, two leaders made a tent-by-tent check on their clients. As they moved toward the last tent, a scream sent them into high gear: "Susie's not breathing!"

Inside the tent, they found the 13-year-old girl not only breathless but also pulseless. They began CPR less than one minute after the initial yell for help. After approximately 10 minutes of ventilations and compressions, Susie gasped for air spontaneously. The rescuers detected a faint pulse. For the next hour, she received periodic artificial respirations to supplement her weak breathing. Around 2:30 AM Susie started to move restlessly and blink her eyes. The storm beat fiercely at the camp for five more hours. The rescuers stayed close to the girl, monitoring her vital signs regularly.

During this time, other members of the group, who knew the area well, hiked out for help. Storm clouds made a helicopter evacuation impossible. Susie was packed in a litter and carried out at approximately 11:00 AM. Although her breathing and heartbeat diminished during the morning, and she lapsed back into a coma, she remained alive, and fully recovered after a three week stay in the local hospital.

Electrophysiology

Lightning occurs most often on hot days when warm, moist air rises rapidly to great heights forming dark clouds filled with static electricity. As a charge accumulates on the bottom of the cloud, an opposite charge develops on the top of the cloud, and on the ground below the cloud. When the difference between charges reaches a potential greater than the ability of the air to insulate, lightning reaches out to equalize the difference.

The bolt of electricity is a direct current that may reach 200 million volts and 300,000 amps, with a temperature as high as 8,000 degrees C. The bolt may reach out over a mile in front of the storm, and move through a channel 8 cm wide.

Lightning flashes out approximately eight million times per day worldwide, or 100 times per second. It can run inside the cloud, cloud-to-cloud, or ground-to-cloud. But the one that hurts people runs cloud-to-ground. Strikes cause more than 1000 injuries to Americans every year, and between 100 and 300 of those injuries will be fatal. Lightning kills more people every year than all other natural disasters combined, usually between May and September, and those who die are usually working or playing outdoors.

Mechanisms of Injury

DIRECT STRIKE. As the name implies, the bolt of lightning hits the victim directly. The victim has usually been associated with a metal object (bicycle, exterior-frame backpack, ice axe).

SPLASH or SIDE FLASH. The lightning strikes something more appealing than the human (trees, shelters), but "splashes" through the air to hit the victim.

GROUND CURRENT. The charge radiates out from the strike point along the ground. This is lightning's most common way of harming people, and the effect may result in many injuries from one strike. Standing or walking with your feet spread creates a "stride potential", and encourages the charge to enter one leg and exit the other. This pathway spares the heart and brain but is not without hazard. The least damage done by a lightning strike occurs with the "flashover" effect, when the charge passes over or around the wet victim without entering their body.

BLAST EFFECT. The explosive expansion of air from the superheat of the lightning produces the thunder, and can produce injuries in a victim who is thrown by the sudden movement of the air.

Types of Injuries

CARDIAC INJURIES. The current of lightning upsets and sometimes stops the natural rhythm of the heart. If the heart is healthy, it often restarts on its own. But it may fail to start up again because it is too damaged or suffering lack of oxygen from . . .

RESPIRATORY INJURIES. The muscles used for breathing have been shut down by the charge of electricity.

NEUROLOGIC INJURIES. The victim is most often knocked unconscious by the charge, and even more will suffer temporary paralysis, especially in the lower extremities. Seizures and/or the inability to remember what happened may result.

BURNS. It is not common to have serious skin and muscle burns after a lightning strike, but superficial, feather-like burn patterns are very common. If the burn is deep and penetrating, the patient usually has much more to worry about than the burn. But treatment for lightning burns is the same as any burn treatment. (See BURNS.)

TRAUMATIC INJURIES. The impact of the blast effect can cause just about any trauma you can imagine: fractures, head injury, spinal injury, dislocations, chest and abdominal injuries.

OTHER INJURIES. Post-lightning strike victims complain most often of ringing in their ears, or loss of hearing, that usually resolves in hours to days without permanent damage. But deafness is not impossible. Ears may bleed. Temporary loss of sight is not unusual, but blindness is rare. Victims often are bothered by insignificant nausea and vomiting for a brief period.

Management

Two factors make treatment of lighting strike victims unique. One is the triage of multiple victims, and the other is the efficacy of CPR. First, in triage (the sorting of patients when a group has been injured), rescuers are taught to give priority to those still alive, and let the dead stay dead. It is the simple rule of "the greatest good for the greatest number". After a lightning strike, the still, silent victims are very often recoverable, and the moaning wounded can wait. Second, CPR done aggressively can bring many, many strike victims back to life since they are often physiologically sound, just shorted out. So keep at it.

Otherwise, the same principles apply. When the scene is safe, check the patient's ABC's. Humans do not store electrical charges, so they are safe to touch immediately. If the primary assessment is OK, go on to vital signs and the hands-on patient exam. Treat injuries as found. Evacuate lightning strike victims even when they seem perfectly well. Problems can show up days later.

Prevention

Avoid likely target areas. Does lightning strike the same place twice? Yes, so avoid places that look like they've been hit before. Does lightning strike water? Yes, the most dangerous place is on or near large bodies of water. Move away during a storm. Does lightning like open areas? Yes, and it will strike the tallest object, which may be you, especially if you're wearing a backpack or riding a bike. Move away from tall objects and metal objects.

Currents of electricity run like currents of water, from high to low, so stay out of wet caves, ditches, and low spots that collect water.

Learn to read weather. A developing storm tends to move very fast. When you see the flash, start counting, one-one thousand, two-one thousand, and so

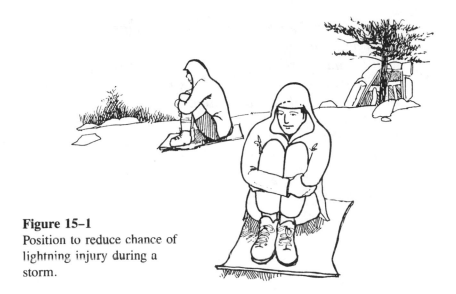

Figure 15–1
Position to reduce chance of
lightning injury during a
storm.

on until you hear the thunder. Sound travels at about one mile per five seconds.
If you get to five-one thousand and hear the roar, you are one mile from the
storm and well within range of the lightning. Seek a safe place before that
happens.

Thick growths of small trees are probably your best bet. Spread out the
group to provide more safety, but make sure everybody can see somebody else.
The lightning can't get everybody that way. Sit on your ensolite pad, or some
other non-conductive object, and make yourself as small as possible. Huddled in
a ball, keeping your feet close together, gives the least potential differences in
the separate points of your body.

Unfortunately, there are no guarantees. Anecdotes indicate that the lightning will get you if it wants you. Be prepared for the worst.

The Barehanded Principles:
Lightning

1. *Avoid dangerous spots.*
   A. *Bodies of water.*
   B. *High and/or open places.*
   C. *Tall objects.*
   D. *Metal objects*
   E. *Low and damp places.*

2. *Spread out the group and make yourself small on an insulating layer.*
3. *If lightning strikes, give the still, silent victim priority treatment, aggressive CPR.*
4. *Check carefully for other injuries.*
5. *Evacuate.*

CHAPTER 16
DROWNING AND NEAR-DROWNING

Introduction

The day was oppressively hot and moist, sultry, and the three high school boys gave up on the fish and dove delightedly into their favorite hole, a cool hollow of water in the woods behind their houses. After the ritual splashing and dunking, two raced for shore. When they looked back, the third was gone.

About six body lengths from shore, turbulence in the still water caught their attention. Swimming back, they found their friend just below the surface, his foot caught in a tangle of submerged roots. They were able to free him, and half-swim, half-drag him to shore. He was not breathing.

While one of the boys pedaled his bike furiously to the nearest phone, calling for help, the other began mouth-to-mouth respirations. Within moments, the victim choked and vomited his lunch across the muddy beach. The ambulance arrived to find all three boys talking excitedly. The ambulance attendants had to convince the victim to go to the hospital for a check up. He never returned home, dying three months later after a series of complicated lung infections.

In recent years, drowning has taken between 6000 and 8000 American lives every year, placing it third as a cause of accidental death. Death results from hypoxia, the lack of air under the water. A near-drowning is a submersion incident in which the victim survives the underwater experience for at least 24 hours, but does not necessarily go on to live a long, healthy life.

Drowning

Management principles don't change just because everybody is wet. Your first concern is safety, which means you must avoid turning yourself or someone else into a second victim in the rescue attempt. Reach to the struggling victim from a secure position. If you can't reach them, with arm or leg or anything extending your reach, throw them something that floats. Or row or paddle out to them. To swim to a struggling, drowning victim is to risk your life. Panic lends them great physical power and determination.

If the drowning victim has been knocked unconscious, attention should be given to the cervical spine, if possible. But not at the exclusion of Airway, Breathing, and Circulation.

Those who die during the submersion go through a series of events that vary little from individual to individual. First, they struggle and fiercely hold their breath. Heart rates speed up and blood pressure rises. Second, the drive to breathe becomes overpowering, and they suck in water. Third, water enters the lungs, and begins crossing cell walls and entering the blood stream. Victims whose lungs are full of water are referred to as "wet" drownings, and they comprise 85–90% of the total drowned victims. (The other 10–15% have "dry" lungs due a constriction of their throat muscles, a laryngospasm, which keeps the water out. These victims go on to die of suffocation.) Fourth, water continues to enter their lungs and their stomachs. They often vomit, and consciousness is lost as they stop trying to breath. Fifth, their oxygen-starved brain begins to suffer. Sixth, their hearts stop, and clinical death occurs. Seventh, the point of irreversible brain damage is reached, biological death.

When the victim is pulled from the water, treatment must begin immediately. Mouth-to-mouth ventilations should start as soon as it is determined there is no breathing. Artificial breathing can even be done while the victim and rescuer are still in the water if the rescuer is stable (for instance, standing in shallows). A victim of laryngospasm will have their airway closed to rescue breathing attempts. If your rescue breaths won't go in, attempt to massage their throat, pushing gently but firmly along their windpipe in order to loosen the spasming muscles.

Once on the shore, determine if the victim's heart is beating. If it isn't, start CPR. Do not worry about the water that may be in their lungs. They are dying from lack of air, and air must be breathed into them. The water in their lungs, remember, is absorbed into their blood. Fresh water submersions have a statistically better chance of survival because the fluid moves more rapidly from the lung to the bloodstream. Salt water may even draw fluid from the blood into the lungs. But rescuers can do nothing about the fluid. They *can* breath vigorously for the victim.

Expect the patient to vomit. When they do, roll them immediately on their side, sweep out the vomitus, roll them back over, and continue CPR. Experts estimate six out of every seven drowned victims are pulled from the aquatic environment soon enough for CPR is be effective if it is started immediately and kept up. It is sobering to consider the dead thousands, mostly children under 14, who could have been saved by trained bystanders.

The duration of the submersion event is obviously a factor in survivability. But the amount of time someone can remain under water, and still recover, is surprising. Especially if they are very young and the water is very cold. Humans, to differing degrees, may experience something akin to the mammalian diving reflex, the physiologic response allowing whales and seals to stay underwater for long periods of time. With submersion in cold water, blood is shunted away from the outside of the body, and concentrated in the heart and lungs and brain, keeping those vital organs alive. In July of 1988, near Salt Lake City, a two-and-a-half year old girl was submerged for approximately 66 minutes in a frigid mountain creek. When found, CPR was started, and continued on route to the hospital. With surgical intervention, she had a 100% recovery!

Near-Drowning

In near-drownings, beware this shunting of blood from the periphery of the body, this aspect of hypothermia that mimics death. It may make pulses too weak to find. Started chest compressions on a cold but beating heart often causes it to stop. So take a much longer time than usual, a minute or more, to check for a pulse before beginning CPR on a cold submersion victim. The patient with a cold, fragile heart should not be handled roughly for the same reason. Breathing for them won't hurt, even if they are doing it for themselves already. Artificial respirations, therefore, should be begun right away if you think they're not breathing.

Near-drowners will probably be hypothermic, and should be treated accord ingly. (See HYPOTHERMIA)

Everyone who has almost drowned should be hurried to a medical facility as soon as possible. It takes very little water in the lungs to have profound effects on the patient. Vital body fluids are washed out, and unhealthy material in the water is absorbed into the body. Pneumonias, tears in weakened lung tissue, chemical imbalances in the blood, and other related problems may result in death days, weeks, or months later.

Prevention

Once again, education is the key. Beware of swimming and diving in unsafe areas. Swim with someone who cares about you, and who knows CPR. Wear a personal flotation device (PFD), and insist on the same from those who accompany you on water-based trips. When crossing rivers on backcountry excursions, chose a safe ford with an open run-out in case you do fall in. Loosen your pack straps before crossing. You might need to shed your gear fast. The difference between an expert and a novice is attention to details.

The Barehanded Principles:
Drowning and Near-Drowning

1. *If needed, start Artificial Respirations as soon as possible.*
2. *Safely remove the victim from the aquatic environment.*
3. *Once on a firm surface, start CPR when there is no pulse.*
4. *Watch the cervical spine, and do a Patient Exam for other injuries.*
5. *Avoid rough handling.*
6. *Treat for hypothermia.*
7. *Evacuate anyone who may have taken fluid into their lungs during the submersion.*

CHAPTER 17
HIGH ALTITUDE ILLNESS

Introduction

A purple human lay stretched across the plaza at Tlamacas Lodge at 12,950 feet above sea level in Mexico. The day before he had been a British Causcasian in Mexico City, and the day before that a pale soldier in the United Kingdom. His pulse rate was 110, and his respirations were 24 and irregular. When we asked him if we could offer some assistance, he told us to "piss off", and vomited violently. We interpreted that as a "yes".

Exchanging pesos for a ride in a car, we took him down to Amecameca, 5000 feet lower. He reported himself much improved the next day, thanked us profusely, and went to a movie.

The medical problems collectively referred to as "altitude illnesses" are the result of hypoxia, insufficient oxygen for normal tissue function. Those who become ill are those too rushed to acclimatize and those who are particularly susceptible. Untreated, the problems can lead to death.

Since there is a measurable increase in ventilations and decrease in aerobic exercise performance above 4000 feet elevation, "high altitude" can be said to start at that point. But complications seldom occur below 10,000 feet, and rarely below 8000 feet. To be safe, consider 8000 to 12,000 feet as high altitude, 12,000 to 18,000 very high altitude, and 18,000 + as extreme high altitude.

The degree of hypoxia a climber at altitude experiences is relative to the barometric pressure. At 18,000 feet the barometer reads one half that of sea level, making the inspired pressure of oxygen also one half. You effectively get 50% less oxygen with each breath.

Acclimatization

Acclimatization is the process of adjusting to lessening barometric pressure. The rate of acclimatization differs with individual physiology, but most people will adjust enough to prevent illness if they spend two to three days in the 8000–12,000 foot range, and not gain more than 1000 feet of sleeping altitude each successive day. For instance, if you slept at 14,000 feet last night, you can climb beyond 15,000 the next day, but you should drop back down to no more than 15,000 to sleep.

The first stage of acclimatization, and our most important means of adjustment, is increasing our ventilations. Heavy breathing increases the oxygen content of the blood, thus getting more oxygen to body tissues. It's OK to pant. In the second stage, our heart rates speed up. Our pulmonary circulation constricts to increase pressure in our arteries to compensate for the decreasing pressure outside. The blood vessels in our brains dilate. After 5–7 days our heart rates return to normal, but the circulatory changes remain. The third stage is a stimulation of bone marrow to produce more red blood cells, which increases the blood's oxygen-carrying capacity. The final stage occurs on a cellular level with capillary density increasing and muscle cells shrinking and mitochondria increasing. These cellular changes get more oxygen into action quicker and easier. Acclimatization is lost at approximately the same rate as it is gained.

Acute Mountain Sickness (AMS)

All altitude illnesses are degrees of the same inability to adjust, and result most often when a group fails to pace themselves to the slowest acclimatizers. AMS is the most common and most mild form of altitude illness. Symptoms can appear in as little as 6 hours after a rapid ascent to an altitude of 8000 feet or more. Headache is the first complaint. Other symptoms include loss of appetite, nausea, lassitude, and unusual fatigue. Vomiting may occur. Skin may become cyanotic (bluish to purplish).

Ataxia is a loss of muscular control leading to difficulty in maintaining balance. It is the single most useful sign indicating the patient is progressing from a mild to a severe form of Acute Mountain Sickness. A simple check for ataxia is called the "tandem walking test"—having the suspect walk a straight line touching the heel of the front boot to the toe of the back boot with each step. If they can't do it, they're ataxic.

Severe forms of altitude illness include High Altitude Pulmonary Edema (HAPE), the most common cause of death among high altitude climbers, and High Altitude Cerebral Edema (HACE). In addition to ataxia, the victim of HAPE develops crackles (gurgling sounds with breathing). Crackles are an indication of fluid (edema) in the lungs (pulmonary system). The sound appears most often in the right side of the chest, and without a stethoscope can sometimes be heard with an ear pressed against the chest wall of the patient. Fluid may build up to the point where the victim suffers respiratory and cardiac arrest.

In the case of HACE the fluid collects around the brain (cerebrum), and the result may be the sudden onset of a severe headache, hallucinations, seizures, unconsciousness, coma, and death.

Some problems can mimic AMS: dehydration, hypothermia, exhaustion, and carbon monoxide (CO) poisoning. Dehydration should respond to fluid intake, hypothermia to rewarming and fluids and food, exhaustion to rest and fluids and food, CO poisoning to fresh air and rest and fluids.

Treatment

Since you can't predict who will deteriorate from mild to severe altitude illness, and at this point the majority of life-threatening mistakes are made, a victim must *stop ascending* until the symptoms resolve. Painkillers for the headache, and anti-emetics (nausea-relievers), may be safely given. But the Important Rule is: DON'T GO UP UNTIL THE SYMPTOMS GO DOWN! In the presence of possible HAPE or HACE, the treatment is IMMEDIATE DESCENT.

In 24–48 hours a healthy person should acclimatize to a given altitude. The dead are almost always among those who broke the Important Rule.

Supplemental oxygen can relieve symptoms and save lives, but it does not replace going down. A common myth concerning bottled oxygen is that a little will do more harm than good. Any amount will help, but probably only for the time it is being used

Acetazolamide (sometimes sold as Diamox), 250 mg twice/day, can stop AMS from growing worse, and often speed up the acclimatization process. It should be started early in the course of the illness. The drug, available in the United States by prescription only, works very effectively as a prevention, increasing breathing which increases arterial oxygen. Acetazolamide works especially well during sleep periods. It is also a diuretic, counteracting fluid retention. If you plan to use the drug as a preventive measure, do so with a doctor's advise.

If the signs include ataxia or an altered mental status, going down can be augmented with dexamethasone (often sold as Decadron). The drug has shown itself to be effective in the treatment of severe problems and should be reserved for that purpose. There is no evidence that it helps in acclimatization or treating pulmonary edema. By prescription only, the recommended dosage is 4 mg every 6 hours.

Prevention

Prevention of Acute Mountain Sickness is best done by staging your ascent. Allowing adequate time for acclimatization increases your safety and enjoyment. Avoid a rapid ascent from sea level to 8000 feet. Instead, spend a night somewhere in the 5000–7000 feet range. Once arriving at 8000–10,000 feet stay two days and two nights before ascending higher to sleep. When going higher, climb no faster than your ability to acclimatize.

Maintain a diet of 70% or greater carbohydrates, and drink enough water to keep your urine very light in color. Carry water and wear clothing appropriate for easy drinking and urination. Avoid respiratory depressants, like sleeping pills and alcohol, especially during the first two or three days.

Physical fitness does not protect you against AMS. Fitter persons are statistically more susceptible, probably because they tend to go up faster. Training is certainly healthy, but if the training is going to prepare you for altitude it has to be done at altitude.

The Barehanded Principles:
Altitude Illness

1. *Go Down.*
2. *Go DOWN.*
3. *GO DOWN.*

CHAPTER 18
SCUBA DIVING INJURIES

Its use is so common many of us have forgotten the word is an acronym for Self-Contained Underwater Breathing Apparatus. SCUBA divers themselves have also become common, enjoying their sport somewhere in every state. What they don't enjoy are the medical problems that sometimes occur as a result of the changing air pressure relative to the depth of the dive.

Air pressure is defined as 1 atmosphere at sea level, and measured at 14.7 pounds per square inch (psi). The density of water produces rapid changes in air pressure as a diver descends. At 33 feet below the sea's surface (or 34 feet in fresh water), the pressure has increased to 29.4 psi, or 2 atmospheres. The rate of increase in pressure is constant, 1 atmosphere for every 33 feet descended.

Decompression Sickness

As the pressure increases, the amount of gas that can be dissolved in the blood and tissues of the diver increases proportionately. At 2 atmospheres, 2 times the oxygen and nitrogen from the bottled air the diver breathes will be distributed to the tissues of the body. Nitrogen cannot be metabolized, and builds up in the cells. On ascent, the gas is diffused out of the tissue.

But problems can occur if the diver ascends too rapidly, or stays down too long. Bubbles of nitrogen can block blood flow and increase pressure on surrounding tissues. The pain of decompression sickness usually starts about one hour after the dive, but can develop up to 12 hours later.

Signs and symptoms may vary in decompression sickness. Pain is the most common complaint. Feeling weak and tired is also common. There may be difficulty breathing, or terrific headaches. Death is rare, but paralysis may result from delayed treatment.

Decompression sickness is sometimes called the "bends". The pain is most often confined to joints in the arms and legs, especially the shoulder and elbow.

"Bending" the joints increases the pain. Patients may complain of partial or complete numbness in their extremities.

Decompression sickness may involve the skin. A burning or itching is followed by blue and purple marbling. When these colors appear, the patient should be considered more serious.

If the sickness involves difficulty breathing and chest pain, the result may be death. If it leaves the diver seeming to have a spinal cord injury, the result may be paralysis.

Lung Expansion Injury

When the pressure on a gas is doubled, the amount of space it takes up is cut in half. When the pressure in decreased, the gas expands, and the expanding gas must be allowed to escape from the diver's lungs on ascent. If the diver breathes normally while heading for the surface, there is no problem. If the diver runs out of air, if equipment fails, if the diver breath-holds, the expanding air may rupture the lungs. When compressed air is held in the lungs, these problem can occur from a depth of as little as four feet.

Torn lungs may produce a pneumothorax (See CHEST INJURIES). Large bubbles of air may enter the bloodstream. Within minutes of ascent these bubbles can enter the brain and cause a stroke-like death. This is the most common cause of diving deaths. The bubbles may enter other places, and produce severe respiratory difficulties, and cardiac failure.

Ear Barotrauma

Pressure-produced injury (barotrauma) from diving is most commonly experienced in the middle ear. Simply squeezing the nose and blowing gently keeps the pressure between middle ear and outer ear balanced for most divers. Sometimes it doesn't work, and the eardrum ruptures or the middle ear bleeds. The complaints are pain in the ear, and sometimes the jaw and neck, dizziness and nausea, and difficulty hearing.

Treatment

Ear injuries usually take care of themselves. Putting medication in the ear without a physician's advice is not a healthy idea. The eardrum may be open. If the problem is severe, have the ear checked. Medication or more dramatic treatment may be necessary.

Decompression sickness or lung injury require more immediate care. If the symptoms seem mild, place divers on their left side with their feet elevated. This position helps keep bubbles out their heart and brain. Giving them fluids to drink, and aspirin may help. Within a half-hour, they should be better. If they don't improve, or if the symptoms are severe, they should be on their way to a doctor, in the same position. Close monitoring is important. CPR may be required.

Divers Alert Network (DAN) at Duke University in Durham, NC, maintains a 24-hour telephone hotline for diving-related emergencies: (919) 684–8111.

CHAPTER 19
BITES AND STINGS

Introduction

The bites and stings humans receive from other animals vary greatly in severity depending on the type of animal, the reason for the attack, and the way the human acts during the confrontation. Despite the variations, similarities in the damage done by bites and stings do exist. And so we can find general principles for the management of the wounds received from wild creatures.

In order of significance, treatment for bites and stings should include 1) stopping serious blood loss, 2) immediate cleaning of the wound against the introduction of whatever microorganisms were living in the mouth that bit or on the body part that stung, and 3) care to reduce the effects of envenomation if the animal was poisonous.

The similarities in animal attacks will also give us some principles for preventing unhealthy confrontations with creatures of the wild places.

Pit Vipers

The scream came from behind a thick bush near Big Creek Trail in Idaho's Frank Church/River of No Return Wilderness. She leaped over the bush and several intervening boulders with surprising grace considering her pants were half down. The snake went the other way, even faster but with more dignity. During eight weeks of traversing a densely populated rattlesnake region our experience was almost always the same. We'd scream, and they'd slither away. The one exception was a couple of tense moments when a large rattler slid into a mini-box canyon in the middle of our path. It started back toward us before realizing the error and returning to the rocky corner in the trail. We gave it plenty of room while passing, and that was that.

Over the past few years the number of venomous snakes attacking humans has averaged about 8000 per year. Of those bitten, no less than nine and no more than fourteen humans have died each year. The dead have almost always been children and the elderly.

99 out of every 100 poisonous snake bites are received from a pit viper (family Crotalidae), the rattlesnakes, copperheads, and water moccasins. The few remaining bites come from North America's only other venomous family, the coral snakes (family Elapidae).

A pit viper's danger comes from two very special teeth, hinged to swing downward at a 90 degree angle from the upper jaw. The jaw opens very, very wide, allowing the venom to be ejected down canals within the fangs, and into a prey's tissue. The amount of venom and the toxicity of the venom determine the danger to the bitten. For instance, the poison of the Mojave Rattlesnake is approximately 44 times more potent that the Southern Copperhead's.

Pit viper venom is generally yellowish, odorless, and slightly sweet to human taste buds. It evolved from the snakes saliva, which makes sense when you remember the purpose is to acquire and utilize food for the snake, not to deal death and destruction to large, inedible mammals who stumble over the low-lying reptiles. The venom attacks the nervous and circulatory systems of the snake's prey. In a mouse this can spell death in a few minutes. How dangerous is this venom to humans? Depends on the age, size, health, and emotional stability of the victim, whether or not they're allergic to the venom, where they were bitten (near vital organs being the most dangerous), how deep the fangs go, how upset the snake is, the species and size of the snake, and the first aid given to the victim. Arizona is the most likely place to die of a snakebite, with Florida, Georgia, Texas, and Alabama filling out the top five.

One rattlesnake bite in four carries no venom. The other three may vary from insignificant to mild to moderate to severe envenomation. Mild envenomations hurt, swell, turn black and blue, and sometimes form a blister at the site. Moderate envenomations adds swelling that moves up the arm or leg toward the heart, numbness, and swollen lymph nodes. A severe envenomation might add big jumps in pulse rates and breathing rates, profound swelling, blurred vision, headache, lightheadedness, sweating, and chills. Death is possible.

Coral Snakes

Coral snake venom seems to be absorbed directly into the blood stream. Symptoms may come on very quickly, the pain changing rapidly to numbness. The bitten extremity tends to swell very little. The victim may become drowsy, weak, and nauseous, and progress to rapid pulse and respirations, convulsions, and death from heart or respiratory failure.

Lizards

Only two lizards, worldwide, are considered venomous enough to end the life of a human. Unfortunately meetings with both are possible in the Southwest. The Gila Monster and the Mexican Beaded Lizard bite when they are picked up or stepped on. They have powerful jaws to compensate for primitive teeth and no means to inject the poison. They lock on while the venom drools into the wound. You may likely be required to heat the underside of their jaw with matches or a lighter to break their grip. There may be a great deal of local swelling and pain.

Treatment

1. *Calm and reassure the patient, putting them physically at rest with the bitten extremity immobilized and kept lower than their heart.*
2. *Remove rings, watches, or anything else that might reduce the circulation if swelling occurs.*
3. *Measure the circumference of the extremity at the site of the bite and at a couple of sites between the bite and the heart, and monitor swelling.*
4. *Apply a wide elastic wrap starting above the wound and wrapping over and beyond the wound. This light constricting band should NOT restrict blood flow. Monitor the circulation beyond the band by checking pulses, skin color, and sensations the patient may complain of (numbness or tingling).*
5. *Evacuate the patient by carrying or going for help to carry them.*
6. *Safely attempt to identify the biting creature.*
7. *Do NOT cut and suck. Mechanical suction (NOT mouth suction) may be valuable if you get there in the first five minutes. Suction should be applied for 30 minutes.*
8. *Do NOT give painkillers unless the patient is very stable, showing no signs of getting worse.*
9. *Do NOT apply ice or immerse the wound in cold water.*
10. *Do NOT give alcohol to drink.*
11. *Do NOT electrically shock the patient.*

Prevention

1. *Don't try to pick up or capture snakes.*
2. *Check places you intend to put your hands and feet before exposing your body part to a bite.*
3. *Gather firewood before dark, or do it carefully while using a flashlight.*
4. *Keep your tent zipped up at night.*
5. *Wear high, thick boots while traveling in snake country.*
6. *When passing a snake, stay out of striking range, which is about one-half their length.*
7. *If you hear the "buzz" of a rattler, freeze, find it with your eyes without moving your head, wait for it to relax the strike position, and back away slowly.*

Figure 19–1
Black Widow.

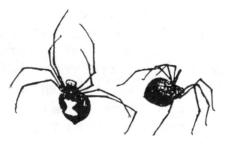

Spiders: Black Widow

About 265,000 per acre! is the answer. How many spiders live in the same forested land we enjoy? is the question. They all love the night. They all have sharp hollow fangs. All but one family have venom glands. They are all strict carnivores.

But very, very few pose a serious threat to humans. One of those is black and beautiful, genus *Lactrodectus,* the shiny female black widow spider. She packs more danger in every drop of venom than any other creature in North America. Fortunately, she is small, reaching a body length usually no more than 18 mm, and more often smaller. Her drop of poison is tiny. The hourglass on her abdomen identifies her.

She has been found in every state but Alaska, privately secluding her web under logs and pieces of bark, in stone crevices, deep in clumps of heavy vegetation. Rarely aggressive, she may be touchy during mating and egg-tending season.

You may not feel the bite. There is little or no redness and swelling at the site. But within 10–60 minutes symptoms begin to occur. Pain and anxiety become intense. Muscular cramping often spreads from the wound, settling in the abdomen and back. Burning or numbness characteristically disturb the victim's feet. Watch for headache, nausea, vomiting, dizziness, and heavy sweating.

You might think you're going to die, but black widows kill only 2–4 people each year, and they are almost always the very young, the very old, or the very allergic.

Keep the victim as calm as possible. That is your best first aid treatment. If you can find the bite site, wash it, and apply an antiseptic like povidone-iodine. Cooling the injury, with ice if possible, with water or wet compresses if necessary, will reduce the pain. Cold also reduces circulation which slows down the spread of the venom.

Evacuation to a medical facility is a great idea, just in case complications arise. Most people will receive painkillers and 8–12 hours of observation. Youngsters and oldsters may be admitted for 24 hours. Antivenin is available if needed.

Undisturbed black widows do not attack humans. Flies are her major source of food. She may consume 2000 insects in her lifetime. Her value to the economy of life is great. Perhaps she deserves less fear, and more respect.

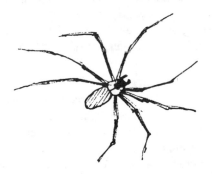

Figure 19–2
Brown Recluse.

Spiders: Brown Recluse

Her name, black widow, is the stuff of nightmares and legends, but the most common serious spider bite in the United States is not from her venom. Instead, look for the secretive brown recluse, genus *Loxosceles*. Generally pale brown to reddish, and 9–14 mm in length, with long slender legs, they most often have the shape of a violin on the front portion of their body. The head of this "fiddle" points toward the tail of the spider. Unlike the black widow, both sexes of Loxosceles are dangerous.

The recluse prefers the dark and dry places of the South and southern Midwest, but travels comfortably in the freight of trucks and trains, and probably can be found in all fifty states. They don't mind the company of humans, and set up web-keeping underneath furniture, within hanging curtains, and in the shadowed corners of closets. Their bite is more common indoors, but they live well-hidden beneath rocks, dead logs, and pieces of bark in forests all over America. They attack more readily in the warmer months, and curious children are their most frequent victims.

Like most spiders, their bite is often painless. Having relatively dull fangs, the serious wounds they inflict are usually on tender areas of the human anatomy. Within 1–5 hours, a painful red blister appears where the fangs did their damage. Watch for the development of a bluish circle around the blister, and a red, irritated circle beyond that. This is the characteristic "bull's-eye" lesion of the brown recluse. The victim may suffer chills, fever, a generalized weakness, and a diffuse rash.

Sometimes the lesion resolves harmlessly over the next week or two. Sometimes it spreads irregularly as an enzyme in the spider's venom destroys the cells of the victim's skin and subcutaneous fat. This ulcerous tissue heals slowly and leaves a lasting scar.

In a few children, death has occurred from severe complications in their circulatory systems.

Without the spider as evidence, it is difficult to be sure what is causing the problem. Initially, there is little to be done other than calming the victim, and applying cold to the site of the bite for reduction of pain. Any "volcanic" skin ulcers should be seen by a physician as soon as possible. The infected area can often be excised, and new skin grafted in with very satisfactory results. Specific medical treatment is now available.

Scorpion

The campfire danced in a pit scooped out of the sand on the banks of the St. Johns River in northern Florida. It gave enough light to add ominously huge shadows to the small scorpion crawling up her arm. She, of course, swept it away. Then screamed in pain. We spent a panicky twenty minutes deciding what to do and loading the canoe for an evacuation. Before the tent was down, her pain was gone with no ill effects. Worldwide, and mostly in warm deserts and semiarid grasslands, live about 650 species of scorpions. They all love the night and hide by day. They all sting with the tip of their "tail", the last few segments of their abdomen. Their pincers are for holding and tearing apart their prey. Insects are their primary source of food.

Most victims report no more pain than a bee sting. An attack of the species *Centruroides* may be different. In North America only the *Centruroides* is a known killer of humans. They are usually straw-yellow or yellow with dark longitudinal stripes, and reach from 2.0 to 7.5 centimeters in length. Their pincers are long and slender as opposed to bulky and lobster-like. The sting is immediately very painful, with the pain increased by a light tap on the site. But resulting deaths have almost exclusively been in small children, the elderly, and the severely allergic. *Centruroides* is only found in Mexico and the extreme southwestern United States.

First aid for any scorpion attack should involve cooling the wound which allows the body to more easily break down the molecular structure of the venom. Cooling also reduces pain. Use ice or cool running water if available. On a warm night, a wet compress will help. And keep the victim calm and still. Panic and activity speed up the venom's spread.

If the scorpion was *Centruroides,* post-sting manifestations may include heavy sweating, difficulty swallowing, blurred vision, loss of bowel control, jerky muscular reflexes, and respiratory distress. These serious signs are cause for quick evacuation to a medical facility. Antitoxins are available in areas where dangerous scorpions live.

In the southwest, most stings occur May through August. The victims are usually putting on clothing, walking barefoot in the dark, or picking up objects (like firewood) off the ground. A bit of forethought can prevent most unfriendly encounters with scorpions.

Ticks

Unable to fly, hop, or leap from overhanging limbs, he waits patiently at the tip of a tall stalk at the side of the trail. His wait might take months. At last, the backpacker brushes past. A relative of the spider, the tick crawls around on his unsuspecting host on eight tiny legs, looking for the right spot to settle down for a few days. He may search for hours. With specialized pincer-like organs, he digs a small wound in his host. Into the wound goes a feeding apparatus called a hypostome, and his relatively powerful sucking mechanism allows him to feed on the blood of the host. Anchored firmly in the wound, he feeds for two to five days, and drops off weighing hundreds of times more than when he first arrived. In the host he often leaves a reminder of his visit, disease-causing microorganisms. Worldwide, only the mosquito spreads more illness than the tick.

Lyme Disease

Beware of the freckle that moves. The comma-sized *Ixodes dammini* tick is stirring up an epidemic of Lyme disease, and an epidemic of hysteria. First diagnosed in Lyme, Connecticut, for unknown reasons the corkscrew-shaped bacteria, a spirochete carried by the tick, has spread to 43 states, still in heaviest concentrations in the Northeast and upper Midwest, and along the coast of northern California.

Experts agree that the panic is unwarranted, but the disease can be scary. And it is the most common tick-borne illness in the United States.

THE WARNING SIGNS:

1) Two days to five weeks after the bite, a well-defined rash appears, a bull's-eye, red surrounded by lighter shades. Unfortunately, about 25% of those infected never get the rash.

2) Flu-like symptoms, with a fever, headache, fatigue, and a stiff neck occur before or after the rash. Rash and illness disappear in a few days to weeks.

3) Extreme, chronic fatigue with irregular heart beat and partial numbness or paralysis can occur weeks to months later. In a few sufferers, this stage can be very serious.

4) Swelling and pain in joints, especially the knees, may start up to two years later. Any joint can be affected, and the arthritis may move from joint to joint with periods of remission.

Lyme is not fatal, although it is possible to die from cardiac complications associated with the disease. But without antibiotic treatment, it can lead to lifelong arthritic problems.

A blood test will show if you have the disease, but only in later stages. Early treatment is recommended based on symptoms if you have been traveling in a known *Ixodes* tick area.

Rocky Mountain Spotted Fever

Montana's Bitteroot Mountains first recorded RMSF, but it has spread from coast to coast. Three to twelve days after the tick has passed the microorganisms, the patient develops a spotty rash, usually beginning on the hands, feet, wrists, and ankles. The spots migrate over the arms, legs, face, and abdomen. Severe headaches are common, with stiff neck and back, and general muscle aches. The characteristic fever rises during the first days, and remains high. If untreated, approximately 20% of the victims will die. Almost everyone will recover with antibiotic treatment.

Colorado Tick Fever

All the Rocky Mountain states have had victims of CTF, as well as western Canada and South Dakota. A virus produces the sudden fever with muscle aches and headache that develops three to six days after the bite of the tick. Diarrhea, vomiting, and stomachaches are common signs and symptoms. The patient often recovers and relapses several times in the course of the illness. It is very rarely fatal, although sufferers report feeling so crummy they wish they could die.

Tularemia

Another bacteria, often borne by ticks of the South and Southwest, causes the high fever and flu-like symptoms of tularemia. A decaying wound at the site of the bite is common. Antibiotics will defeat the bacteria.

Getting Ticked Off

Quick tick removal is necessary since the critter may be latched on 12–24 hours before passing disease-causing bacteria. Forget those ineffective and possibly dangerous ways of smearing them with petroleum jelly, nail polish, or gasoline, or burning them out with a match. Using bare fingers to pull them out works, but it's not the best way. You can crush the tick, propelling their juices into you. A pair of tweezers should be in your first aid kit. If the tweezers are fine-pointed, all the better. Grab the tick near your skin and pull out gently. A piece of your skin may harmlessly pull away with the tick. Dabbing on alcohol before and after makes the job cleaner. No twisting, yanking, or squeezing. Then wash the area thoroughly. Save the tick, preferably without touching it with your hand, if you would like to have it checked for disease. Make note of the time and your location to keep with the removed tick.

A Repelling Thought

Deet (n, n-diethyltoluamide) still works when applied to your skin, but a new repellent keeps ticks from even getting on your clothing. The ingredient is permethrin. Unlike deet, permethrin is sprayed directly on clothing instead of skin, and therefore reduces the chances of the adverse reactions common in high concentrations of deet.

DEET WARNING: Don't put it on infants and small children. Apply it sparingly. Don't use it repeatedly over long periods of time. Use lower concentrations. It is a proven carcinogen in lab tests.

Non-chemical means of tick avoidance are still useful. Wear long pants and shirts with long sleeves. Lighter colors make ticks easier to spot. Tuck pants into socks. Stay near the middle of established trails. Have someone check you carefully for ticks a couple of times each day on a backcountry trip or after any jaunt into known tick areas.

Rabies

Dawn brought a storm of unprecedented fury to an isolated Iranian village in the mid-1970's. Contact with the outside world was cut off. Driven by wind and floods of water, a pack of seven wolves from neighboring hills entered the village. At least 73 of the Iranians were significantly bitten, obvious typical tearing canine wounds. Peace Corps volunteers treated the wounds but were helplessly without vaccination against rabies. All seven of the wolves were eventually killed, and all were tested positive for the rabies virus.

Of the 73 injured villagers, 30, or approximately 40%, developed rabies and died. The remainder, even though they received similar bites, failed to develop the virus.

From this, and other evidence, researchers have concluded that you have a 4-in-10 chance of developing rabies even if you are bitten by a rabid animal. This doesn't mean you should take the chance of not being treated. Rabies is a 100% fatal disease once the virus sets up housekeeping in a human brain. The only survivors of rabies are those few people who have received specific medication before the virus reached their medulla.

Annually in the U.S. about one million people are treated for animal bites, including those inflicted by other humans. 20–25,000 of these people will be treated for rabies. Each year somewhere between 0 and 3 cases of human rabies will actually be diagnosed, and those diagnosis will be made postmortem (after death). In December, 1987, the only case of human rabies in the last three and a half years showed up in San Francisco in a 13-year-old male. Your chance of being hit by a meteor is better than your chance of contracting rabies.

Statistics from the United States, Canada, and Mexico give us the primary reservoirs of rabies. The major hosts are skunks (43%), followed by raccoons (28%), bats (14%), cattle (4.6%), cats (3%), and dogs (1.7%). The rest of the carriers were a few wolves, bobcats, coyotes, groundhogs, muskrats, weasels, woodchucks, foxes, horses, and a rare human. The significant stat for outdoor enthusiasts to note in 96% of the rabies in the U.S. is carried by wild animals.

Only mammals get rabies, and it acts in this way: the virus travels at a constant speed from the bite site to the spinal cord, and up the cord to the medulla where it replicates and demands the death sentence. It then travels back out along the nervous system. The animal becomes infectious after the rabies virus collects in the saliva glands. It is transmitted to other mammals through bites that tear the flesh. The incubation period in humans, the time from bite to brain, varies with individuals and with the bite site. Ten days is the minimum, and one year the maximum. An average individual would incubate the virus for about three weeks after a bite on the face, and about seven weeks after a bite on the foot.

Infected animals can spread the disease without biting. If their saliva contacts a mucous membrane (the inner surface of lips or the eye) or an already open wound, the disease may result. There are several well-documented cases of transmission by corneal transplant.

Rabies produces general early signs and symptoms: headache and fever, cough and sorethroat, loss of appetite and fatigue, abdominal pain, nausea, vomiting, diarrhea. Once in the central nervous system the virus makes the victim anxious, irritable, depressed, disoriented, unable to sleep, and prone to hallucinations. They may complain of stiff neck, double vision, and visual sensitivity to light. You may notice muscle twitching and, later, seizures. The final stage includes bizarre behavior like aimless unreasonable activity, biting at those who approach, and drooling. Painful muscle spasms in the throat result when the victim tries to eat or drink. The pain leads to avoidance of swallowing, and thus drooling. Some victims will have throat spasms at the sight of water, and so the name "hydrophobia" (fear of water) became attached to rabies. As the nervous system deteriorates, victims become paralyzed, slip into a coma, and die. Life after rabies is brief and very unpleasant.

Treatment

Immediate care for the bite of any animal, including rabid animals, needs to concentrate on cleaning the wound. Scrub it vigorously. Wash it with soap if you have any available. Scrub in iodine or alcohol if you have any. Rinse the wound thoroughly. Iodine, alcohol, and some detergents will kill the rabies virus. The sooner cleaning takes place, the better.

As soon as possible, have the wound checked by a physician. Tetanus or antibiotics may be recommended to prevent bacterial infections. The doctor might suggest you have the rabies vaccine. Fortunately the current Human Diploid Cell Vaccine against rabies works every time. A series of five shots goes into your arm instead of the old painful abdominal injections. To be most effective, the shots should be started within 72 hours of the bite.

When to be Treated

How do you decide if the animal whose bite you carry had rabies? There is only one sure way: have the brain of the animal tested for presence of the virus. This is often impossible. Without the head, five other questions should be asked. 1) Was the animal one of the highly suspect species? 2) Was the attack provoked? Rabid animals tend to attack without provocation. (Trying to pick up or feed a wild animal and having it take a nip out of your finger is a very natural and unsuspect action. Having it leap from the shadows at your throat is an unprovoked and suspect attack.) 3) If the animal was a pet, what is its vaccination status? 4) What is the geographical incidence of rabies in the area of the attack? And most importantly, 5) How did the animal behave in general? Loss of natural timidity and weird behavior are the surest non-clinical signs of rabies infection in animals.

When in doubt, get the expensive shots. If you make the wrong choice, you have accepted the death sentence.

CHAPTER 20
BEAR ATTACKS

Dropped by helicopter in the Yukon-Tanara region of eastern Alaska, Cynthia began to gather rock samples as her job required. Minutes later she was surprised by a bear. Despite her yelling and backing away, the bear approached, and suddenly attacked. Cynthia was thrown to the ground where she played dead. The bear continued its attack, severely biting her right shoulder, upper arm, head, and neck. After several minutes of mauling, it dragged her downslope a short distance.

When the bear stopped for a rest, Cynthia, in an act of supreme self-control, keyed her radio and called quietly to the helicopter for help. Hearing her, the bear renewed the attack, removing all the muscle from her upper left arm.

Sensing the bear intended to eat her, Cynthia began to struggle as fiercely as she could, screaming and kicking at the bear. It backed off, and moved to her backpack, tearing into her food. For approximately ten more minutes, she lay still and watched the bear. When the helicopter finally returned, the bear left the area.

A brave and strong woman, Cynthia recovered, but her injuries required the removal of both her arms. The bear was never located. It had been a medium-sized black bear.

Encounters with Bears

Encounters with bears are always potentially dangerous. They are powerful meat-eaters, and we are weak meat. Although bears are unpredictable at best, historical evidence gives specific guidelines for reducing the risk of the encounters being harmful or fatal to humans.

1. Keeping your face toward the bear, back away slowly and quietly. Running makes you a high profile target that may attract the bear out of curiosity if nothing else.

2. Slowly loosen back straps and waistbelts, in case you need to drop them.

3. Look around slowly for trees that may be climbable, but keep in mind a hungry bear will climb a tree almost as fast as it runs.

4. When you have lost sight of the bear, move downwind and away while keeping an eye open for the bear.

5. If the bear charges, drop your pack and continue backing away slowly. It may be bluffing, or it may be distracted by the pack.

6. If the bear is a solitary black, and it attacks, scream and fight back, using a weapon if possible.

7. If the bear has cubs, if the bear is a grizzly, roll into a ball, pull your chin to your chest, clasp your hands behind your neck, make no sound, and play dead.

Prevention of Bear Encounters

1. In bear country, keep to wide trails or open country, avoiding a surprise meeting.

2. Make noise while you travel, especially sounds ranging from high to low, like singing and yelling. (Little dingling bells on your pack are of marginal use.)

3. Travel in a group. Bears rarely attack a group of four or more.

4. Avoid traveling in the dark.

5. Camp away from obvious bear sign (tracks, scat, scratches) and active game trails.

6. Loop a rope over a high limb and hoist your food above a bear's reach (above the ground and away from the trunk of the tree), at least 100 yards from camp, and downwind. Consider toothpaste, deodorants, or anything attractively fragrant as food.

7. Avoid smelly, greasy foods like bacon, sausage, and fish.

8. Sleep in a tent, and bring nothing inside that might attract a bear.

9. Cook away from your tent. Keep your camp clean, hanging your trash with your food, washing cookware.

10. Leave your dog at home. Bears have been known to chase dogs back to their owners, and they arrive already upset.

11. During their menstrual period, women should consider staying out of bear country.

12. Human sexual activity seems to attract bears.

13. Aerosol sprays containing capsicum, a derivative of red pepper, will often repel bears if you can give them a blast in the face.

14. Where permissible, it might be wise to carry a gun. It should be a big gun.

When the Bear Bites

Bears are capable of removing significant portions of a victim's body, and leaving a high risk of infection. Of first priority is stopping bleeding (See SOFT TISSUE INJURIES). If rapid evacuation to medical attention is not available, scrub the wound clean, using an iodine solution of not more than 5%. Cover the wound with a sterile dressing, and immobilize the bitten area. Evacuate as speedily as possible.

CHAPTER 21
DANGEROUS MARINE LIFE

Early morning, Christmas Day, 1984. The missing surfer, a loner, was found dead, his body rolling in the waves of an isolated northern California beach. He still wore what remained of his black neoprene wetsuit. A bite wound extended from his left armpit to just above his left hip, twenty-eight inches across. Gone from his chest and abdominal cavities were the left side of his rib cage, his left lung, diaphragm, stomach, left kidney, and parts of his liver and intestines. Only one fish on earth, said the experts from the Monterey Bay Aquarium, was capable of such a large bite—the great white shark. This one, they estimated, had been twenty-two feet long, and weighed over one ton.

Below the dancing surface of the ocean, which covers about seventy-one percent of the earth, live four-fifths of the world's organisms. Some of these creatures are potentially dangerous to humans. Generally, risky aquatic life can be divided into three categories: 1) those with big teeth, 2) those that envenomate, and 3) those that sting with nematocysts.

Those with Big Teeth

Of all fish worldwide, sharks elicit the greatest fear. And deservedly so. Their triangular teeth are continually migrating forward to fall out and be replaced by new ones growing in the back of their crescent-shaped mouths. The result is an orifice always full of razor-keen weapons capable of removing large amounts of tissue from a prey's body. They account for the most human deaths annually from aggressive marine life. Even so, the number of shark attacks each year averages only between fifty and one hundred in all the seas of earth. It seems safe to go back in the water considering the ratio of sharks to people who swim off shore.

If you work or play in the oceans of the United States, your chance of being shark food is perhaps one in five million. There are steps you can take to reduce the risk of attack even more: 1) Swim in groups. 2) Do not swim at dusk or during the night in infested waters. Those are the times sharks feed. 3) Wear bright or gaudy-colored swimsuits or wetsuits that reduce the chance of being mistaken for something sharks like to eat. 4) Avoid turbid water where the shark's eyesight will be impaired. 5) Avoid thrashings and splashing and other erratic movements and noises that attract attention. Sharks hunt with vibration-receptors as well as their eyes. 6) Be watchful if you are a successful spear-fisher. Sharks also use their sense of smell, and are attracted to blood and other body fluids in the water.

If a shark seems interested in you, face it and swim away slowly. Avoid the crawl stroke, the butterfly, and other quick swimming styles. Stick to a breast stroke or easy side stroke. If the shark charges, curl into a ball. If it seems intent on taking a bite out of you, kick and punch at the eyes, nose, and gills.

In warmer waters, swimmers sometimes run the risk of toothy contact with barracudas or moray eels. Barracudas seldom attack humans, but when they do it is swift and fierce, and usually in murky water where they have become confused. Their big V-shaped mouths, with long pointed teeth, can do much damage. The glitter of shiny paraphernalia, and jerky swimming movements, may attract the barracuda. Moray eels do not bite unless threatened. Their sharp teeth and powerful jaws tend to hold a victim so strongly that the eel has to be killed to be removed. Divers are at risk if they stick their hands into coral holes and rock crevices where eels like to lurk in wait for tastier morsels than humans.

Those that Envenomate

With the exception of sea snakes, venomous sea creatures are non-aggressive organisms that are stepped on or handled unknowingly. The most likely of these animals to become the victims of human carelessness are sting-rays and sea urchins. Contact usually produces local burning pain, followed by redness, swelling, and aching (and bleeding in the case of the stingray who has large barbs on the end of its tail).

The wound should be cleaned immediately with sea water. Explore the clean wound and remove any loose piece of the creature that may be stuck in the patient. Cleaning will also remove some of the venom, and, if the water is cold, relieve some of the initial pain. Scrubbing the wound with a povidone-iodine solution can help reduce the effects of the venom. As soon as possible, soak the wound in hot water. This may further remove venom. Once the early pain has eased, the application of heat should not increase it. Check again for debris in the wound. These injuries carry a high risk of infection. When the wound has dried, cover it with a sterile dressing and bandage it loosely. With all marine-related cuts, a loose bandage is best, allowing the wound to drain. Monitor the patient for signs of infection, an indication a doctor is needed. (See INFEC-TION).

Hawaii is the only State with sea snakes. Reptiles in every sense of the word, they breathe air but can remain submerged for hours. Commonly ranging from three to four feet in length, individuals have been measured to nine feet. They flatten out toward the rear, and propel themselves forward and backward with undulating motions, like delicate ribbons waving in sea currents. Attacks are rare, unless they are provoked. Their short fangs deliver a relatively mild bite. But the venom is very toxic.

Developing in minutes to hours, the patient complains of nausea and non-specific feelings of illness. Their level of anxiety increases. Pain grows, with partial paralysis possible. Difficulty breathing may follow. Heavily envenomated patients develop a growing intensity of signs and symptoms, and may lapse into a coma. One in four victims die without antitoxin.

Treatment in the field consists of removing the patient from the water, and calming them. Hysteria and movement increase the activity of the poison. Place a light constricting band, not a tourniquet, close to the bite and between the wound and the patient's heart. Cutting and sucking is dangerous and non-productive. Evacuate the patient as soon as possible to a medical facility.

Those with Nematocysts

Coelenterates form an enormous phylum of sea creatures with around 9000 named species. Some of them are harmful to humans, with common names that sometimes reflect the risk they pose: fire coral, stinging medusa, Portuguese man-of-war, sea wasp, sea nettle, hairy stinger, stinging anemone. They all share a stinging organelle, called a nematocyst, that lives encapsulated in a cnidoblast on the tentacles of the coelenterate. The cnidoblast has a trap door (the operculum) with a trigger (the cnidocil) that opens the door. Filled with venom, the nematocyst has a sharp, coiled, thread-like appendage which springs out when the trigger is touched, lodging in the victim.

The reaction in humans will range from mild to severe. Mild reactions are immediate, and include stinging, burning, itching, and sometimes local numbness to touch. The stung area may acquire a bruised appearance that lingers for days. A moderate reaction progresses to headache, nausea, and vomiting. Severely reactive victims have difficulty breathing that may lead to loss of consciousness, convulsions, and the possibility of death.

Since the leading cause of death is drowning in the ensuing panic, removal of the victim from the aquatic environment is of immediate importance. Once safely out of the water, the irritated area of the victim's skin should be rinsed with sea water. Rinsing with fresh water may stimulate the nematocysts that have not fired to do so. Physically lift off any tentacles that still cling to the patient, but do so without touching the tentacles with a naked hand. The organelles that aren't rinsed off should be "fixed" so they will cease to envenomate. A wash of alcohol will work. Ammonia, vinegar, and urine have been used successfully. Meat tenderizer, mixed with one of the liquids to form a paste, and applied to the skin, is an effective fixer. Keep the fixer on until the pain goes away. It might take as long as a half hour.

The final step in treatment is to remove the embedded nematocysts. They can be rubbed off with sand and sea water, shaved off with a knife, or scraped off gently with anything that has an appropriate edge.

Persistent itching can be relieved with a corticosteroid cream from the first aid kit. The patient should be watched over the next 24 hours for signs of a severe allergic reaction. (See ANAPHYLAXIS).

CHAPTER 22
MEDICAL EMERGENCIES

Introduction

Little Jimmy stopped dipping his paddle uselessly into the Wekiva River and turned to me from the bow of the canoe.

"I can't do this any more," he groaned.

Knowing he hadn't been doing anything to move us toward our campsite for the last hour, I swallowed my impatience and asked, "Why not?"

Jimmy's reply was, "My kidneys hurt. I think they're failing."

One has a very short life expectancy, a couple of hours maybe, after one's kidneys fail! "How do you know it's your kidneys?"

"It happened last year about this time," said Jimmy.

"Tell me," I asked compassionately, "where it hurts."

Jimmy's trembling hand swept broadly over his entire lower torso. "Right here, in my kidneys."

I knew immediately that he was either 1) lying, 2) mistaken, or 3) an anatomical marvel.

"Lie back against the cargo and give your kidneys a rest," I suggested.

Sometimes my medical astuteness amazes even me. By the time we reached our camp, Jimmy had made an astounding 100% recovery.

Sometimes the emergencies you face in the backcountry will not be caused by an injury, but by an illness (or by a supposed illness). The pain, discomfort, weakness, distress your patient feels will be the result of a non-injury variation from the way they normally function. Your job is to figure why they're dysfunctioning, and how you can help them.

125

Assessment

Your primary concerns are still the same as with an injury: the ABC's. Checking and re-checking the Vital Signs are still the important ways to tell how your patient is doing. (See PATIENT ASSESSMENT). Your Patient Exam may be revealing.

The History you take will be the critical determining factor in your assessment. It is worth repeating the PQRST questions:

PROVOKES. Does anything provoke the pain and discomfort? Movement? Body position? Touching a certain spot?

QUALITY. Ask the patient to describe the sensation. Is it sharp and stabbing? A dull ache? A squeezing pressure?

RADIATION. Does the pain have a specific location, and does it radiate from there? Or is the discomfort generalized?

SEVERITY. Ask the patient to rate the pain on a scale of one-to-ten with ten being the worst imaginable torment. Their answer will be important, but their answer an hour later will be even more important as an indicator of their well-being.

TIME. How long has the problem been going on?

The AMPLE survey can be equally important in your gathering of historical clues. Are they ALLERGIC to anything they know of? Are they taking any MEDICATIONS (legal or otherwise)? Is there any relevant PAST ILLNESS (has this happened before)? When (and what) was their LAST MEAL? What were the EVENTS that led up to this episode?

CHAPTER 23
ACUTE ABDOMEN

There are a great number of things that can go wrong in the abdominal cavity. Some of the disorders can cause death in a short time without surgical intervention. It is not necessary to figure out what is going wrong. It *is* necessary to know that something serious is happening. That something serious is termed an "acute abdomen".

The patient often first reports a "stomachache", one of the more common backcountry complaints. Many of these problems are not serious, and can be treated successfully or left to resolve on their own. The patient with an acute abdomen will present differently. During your examination, check for distention of the abdominal wall and a tenderness in a specific area. With your ear pressed against the abdomen listen for at least a full minute for sounds of bowel activity. Growing rigidity and distention, specific tenderness, and the absence of bowel sounds are very unhealthy signs. A fever with a prolonged stomachache is cause for a high level of concern. The presence of blood as 1) pink to red color in the urine, 2) black "tar" in the stool, or 3) "coffee grounds" in the vomitus is reason for alarm. They like to vomit. When kidneys are functioning improperly, a pain response can usually be elicited by tapping over their position, where the last ribs join the backbone.

Answers to the PQRST questions will round out your assessment. Pain is often Provoked by lying flat, and eased by sitting or lying with legs curled up. The Quality of the pain increases in sharpness. The pain may Radiate from an unhealthy spleen to the left shoulder, from a clogged gall bladder to right shoulder, from the stomach toward the appendix with appendicitis, and it tends toward a specific focus rather than a general discomfort. The Severity increases. If the Time involved is more than twenty-four hours, or more than eight hours without diarrhea, you should be on your way to a medical facility.

Treatment

Keep the patient calm and lying down in the position most comfortable for them. Keep them warm, and monitor their condition for signs of shock (see SHOCK). Give them nothing by mouth unless a long evacuation creates the risk of dehydration in which case you might give them small sips of cold water. They need a hospital as rapidly as possible. The evacuation should be as gentle as you can make it. Jarring usually causes a great deal of pain for the acute abdomen.

The Barehanded Principles:
Acute Abdomen

1. *Watch for specific, burning, enduring pain with a fever and/or blood in the urine, stool, or vomit.*
2. *Keep them in their most comfortable position.*
3. *Keep them warm.*
4. *Treat for shock, should it develop.*
5. *Evacuate gently as soon as possible.*

CHAPTER 24
ANAPHYLAXIS

Once again the sun was high, and the days were long. We were easing ourselves into another summer season. For most outdoor adventurers this is a time when backcountry travel becomes simplified. You don't have to carry as much warm clothing or heavy winter equipment, nature is less hostile, and the perils of being in wild places seem non-existent. For a few, this is not the case. Instead summer is associated with anxiety over an attack by a stinging insect, and the possibility of anaphylaxis.

Jan is one of those who worries. Last summer, Jan and her friend Mark were out on a week-long hike through a New England wilderness area. The weather was fine, and the hiking spectacular. But in mid-afternoon of the fourth day, they stopped for a break, and set their packs on a ground hornet's nest. Before they realized their mistake, both had been stung.

Mark and Jan had been stung before. Mark had the typical reaction: a painful, raised welt that cleared up over approximately 24 hours. Jan, on the other hand, knew that she was now in a life-threatening situation. She was allergic to the venom. When she had been exposed to proteins in the venom in the past, she developed a "hypersensitivity reaction" to them.

Within our bodies are a series of White Blood Cells which are constantly on the lookout for invaders. In order to do this, these cells must be able to distinguish between "self" and "non-self", so our own WBC's don't attack us! WBC's attack and destroy invading *foreign* protein. In the process they develop a "memory" of the invader so they can mobilize defense forces more quickly in the future. These additional forces are called in through the release of a chemical called histamine, released from our MAST cells.

In Mark's case, just enough histamine is released. Jan, a hypersensitive, released far too much histamine. Her immunological system over-reacted. But why is this a threat to her life?

Histamine not only helps call in reinforcements. It also causes itching. It is a very powerful vasodilator, opening blood vessels up wide. Histamine is an equally powerful bronchoconstrictor, causing airways to close down.

Jan's anaphylactic reaction turns her skin red within minutes. She develops itchy hives. She has difficulty breathing, and it gets worse. Without immediate care, Jan's airway may shut completely, and she may die of asphyxiation.

The best compound known that will reverse the effect of the histamine is epinephrine (adrenalin). Jan carries it in her Bee Sting Kit, and both she and Mark know how to use the kit.

Jan ran down the trail to avoid more stings. Mark grabbed her pack and dug out the kit from a handy side pocket. Though some kits are spring-loaded, Jan's requires a manual injection. Inside are a complete set of printed instructions, but they must be read before a crisis. No time for reading now! Removing the rubber cover from the needle, Mark grasps the back of Jan's upper arm where it meets her shoulder. He darts the needle in at a 45 degree angle, as far as it will go. Pulling back slightly on the plunger, he checks to see if blood is drawn into the syringe, indicating he has hit a vein. (It he hits a vein, he will withdraw the needle, and insert it again.) He pushes down on the plunger as far as it will go. Withdrawing the needle, he massages Jan's arm to speed the drug into circulation.

In moments, Jan can breathe easier. She takes the four antihistamine tablets that came in her kit. These usually take 30-40 minutes to be absorbed into the body. The epinephrine will last about 20-30 minutes. Occasionally the anaphylactic state will return before the tablets take effect. But Jan's kit has a second injection of epinephrine should she need it.

Jan's case is not uncommon, and ground hornets are not the only danger. Any foreign protein finding its way into a human can create problems. People are often allergic to bees, wasps, yellow jackets, ants, black flies, and some foods and drugs. As result they carry an Anakit (or Bee Sting Kit).

One concern often voiced is: Is it legal to give someone an injection? Yes, if it's their kit. But if it's your kit, and you recognize the inability to breathe indicating a severe anaphylactic reaction in someone else, err on the side of conservation of life.

The Barehanded Principles:
Anaphylaxis

1. *Before a backcountry trip starts, learn if any-one if the group is hypersensitive to any known substances.*

2. *Carry a Bee Sting Kit, and know how to use it.*

3. *Ready the kit if a known hypersensitive con-tacts the allergen they are hypersensitive to.*
4. *Keep them calm.*
5. *Give them the antihistamine tablets if they can swallow.*
6. *Give them the injection if they cannot breathe.*
7. *If the injection is given, evacuate the patient, even if they appear to be fully recovered.*

CHAPTER 25
DIABETES MELLITUS

Carbohydrates and some proteins are converted into glucose during diges-
tion. Glucose is the main source of energy for the cells of the human body.
Some parts of the body (muscles, fat, the liver) store glucose for future need.
Some parts, especially the brain, cannot store glucose in significant amounts. To
meet the needs of the brain, we carry sugar in our blood at all times. Islet cells
of the pancreas form insulin, a hormone necessary for glucose to be utilized.
Without it, blood sugar circulates but cannot be absorbed by cells. Diabetes is a
disease characterized by a pancreas that produces an insufficient amount of
insulin.

Sometimes the insufficiency of insulin production is complete, and the patient must inject the hormone into their bodies on a daily basis. This is often
referred to as Type I, or insulin-dependent diabetes. Sometimes the insufficiency is partial, and the patient can control their disease with diet and exercise.
They may require an oral medication to stimulate insulin production. This is
referred to as Type II, or non-insulin-dependent diabetes. Either patient may be
able to regulate their disease and lead an active life, traveling far into the backcountry. The diabetic who may need your care is one who is suffering from
hypoglycemia (low blood sugar) or hyperglycemia (high blood sugar). Hypoglycemia, or insulin shock, is more common.

Hypoglycemia

Blood sugar levels can drop to dangerously low levels in the diabetic who
exercises too much, eats too little, or takes too much insulin. Because of the
brain's dependency on glucose in the blood, hypoglycemia can quickly lead to
unconsciousness, permanent brain damage, and death.

The first sign is usually an altered level of consciousness, confusion, irritability, and restlessness. Their skin tends to be pale and sweaty. Their pulse is rapid. They often complain of hunger, headache, dizziness, and weakness. These signs and symptoms can mimic alcohol intoxication. The problem usually develops rapidly, and may lead to convulsions and coma.

If recognized soon, while they can still swallow, the patient needs a sugary liquid or another concentrated sweet source (maybe candy or syrup). Commercially made glucose preparations are advisable additions to the first aid kit of anyone traveling with a diabetic. If the patient is having difficulty swallowing, the concentrated glucose can be squeezed between the cheek and gum where gulping it down will be a reflex action.

As soon as the patient has regained a more stable level of consciousness, they should be given more solid food and encouraged to rest for several hours before continuing.

If the patient is unconscious, maintenance of the airway should take immediate precedence. Roll them into the recovery position, on their side, which allows for drainage of any fluids from the mouth while keeping their tongue forward and away from their airway. Rub syrup, honey, sugar, or a high glucose concentrate from the first aid kit, into their cheek and gum. Keep at it until they recover enough to feed themselves. A patient who is slow to recover, or who fails to recover completely, should be evacuated for medical attention.

Any victim unconscious for unknown reasons should be considered a possible diabetic. Check quickly for medic alert tags or wallet cards. Question bystanders. Even without evidence, sugar can be administered safely.

Hyperglycemia

High blood sugar can result from too little exercise, too much food, or too little insulin. A diabetic who is sick for another reason may develop hyperglycemia due to changes in insulin requirements brought on by the other illness. Though not immediately dangerous, blood sugar levels creeping up over a period of days leads to increased urination as the kidneys work overtime expelling the excess sugar. Lost with the sugar are water and electrolytes, and dehydration commonly results. Untreated, the dehydration and inadequate energy supply can lead to impaired mental function, coma, and death.

The typical slow onset of this diabetic coma is characterized by growing irritability and confusion. Deep respirations (air hunger) with a fruity breath odor are common. The patient's skin becomes warm, dry, and flushed. They usually complain of headache, intense thirst, nausea, stomachache, and the need to frequently urinate.

Diabetic coma is not common because the patient usually notices the slow changes in their condition and takes steps to reverse their deterioration. If they are taking the right steps and improvement does not result, they should be evacuated as soon as possible for insulin therapy. Unconsciousness due to hyper-glycemia requires a physician with all haste.

Sometimes you may not know if the unconscious diabetic is hypoglycemic or hyperglycemic. In that case treat hypoglycemia. Sugar may save the victim of insulin shock and it won't harm the victim of diabetic coma.

The Barehanded Principles:
Diabetes

1. *Ensure an adequate diet with plenty of fluids is available for the diabetic before the backcountry trip begins.*
2. *Extra insulin should be carried in the backcountry, and not all of it in one pack or canoe in case of loss.*
3. *High and low temperatures can ruin insulin. It might need to be carried in a temperature controlled package such as a thermos.*
4. *As many people as possible should know the needs of the diabetic, where the insulin is kept, and how to administer it.*
5. *Encourage the diabetic to balance exercise with food and insulin intake.*
6. *Diabetes affects the circulation of the patient putting them at high risk for infection from superficial wounds. Check regularly for small cuts and abrasions.*
7. *The same lack of circulation makes a diabetic prone to frostbite. Protect accordingly.*
8. *Any alteration in the level of consciousness of the diabetic should be investigated immediately.*
9. *Administer sugar for hypoglycemia, or if in doubt as to the cause.*
10. *Evacuate anyone who does not show early signs of recovery.*

CHAPTER 26
POISONING

Any substance a person eats, breathes, absorbs, or gets injected into their body can cause a malfunction in normal metabolic activity. The substance is then called a poison. Most of the deaths from poisoning occur in homes to small children. In the backcountry fatal poisonings are rare. When they do happen, it's usually the result of an inadequately ventilated tent or snowcave that lets carbon monoxide build up, the ingestion of a deadly plant or fungus, or injection of venom by a dangerous animal (See BITES AND STINGS). Giving the patient proper care requires you to first identify the problem, and second identify the offending substance.

Inhalation

Stoves burn inefficiently in an enclosed space with inadequate oxygen. Higher altitudes increase the chance of poor combustion. The result of incomplete combustion is carbon monoxide (CO). CO is invisible and odorless, and once inhaled, it enters the blood of the victim where it is about 200 times more bondable to the hemoglobin. Hemoglobin normally carries oxygen out to the cells of the body. With CO attached, hemoglobin is now useless. Tissue death can occur rapidly, and lead to the death of the organism.

As the amount of attached carbon monoxide increases, the patient's level of consciousness descends into irritability, impaired judgment, and confusion. They'll develop a terrible headache, loss of visual acuity, dizziness, and nausea. It will be increasingly difficult for them to get a full breath. Toward the end, their skin will turn red, their heart will fail, and they will die.

Being careful of your own safety, move the patient to fresh air. If they have been exposed to low concentrations of CO, they'll probably recover completely in a few hours. If the concentrations have been high, they may die even removed from the source of the gas. They need rapid evacuation to a pressure chamber and high concentrations of supplemental oxygen. An unconscious victim of CO poisoning will need to have their airway maintained during the evacuation.

Ingestion

Swallowed poisons can disturb the body's balance in many, many different ways, and you may find it impossible to discover the cause of your patient's distress.

In general it would be a healthy idea to become wary of any change in the level of consciousness of a suspected poison victim. Ask about nausea and vomiting, abdominal cramps, diarrhea, loss of visual acuity, muscle cramps, or anything else unusual. Watch for signs of shock.

The historical evidence you gather will be most helpful in assessing the problem. What have they put into their mouth in the last 24 hours? When did they do it? How much did they eat? If more than one person suffers, what have they consumed in common? If they're unconscious, what is lying around that could have poisoned them? Ask about underlying medical problems that could be simulating a poisoning.

If your level of suspicion is high, start treatment quickly. Each moment that passes lets more and more poison be absorbed into your patient's system. It would be nice to have a Backcountry Poison Control Center to call. They could provide immediate and exact information to guide you. In their absence, you are left with some management principles.

If they are unconscious, try to find out what could have poisoned them and carry out a sample. But evacuation to a medical facility is probably what is going to save them. Keep them on their side to maintain their airway.

If they are conscious, inducing vomiting may be very beneficial. Emetics are vomiting-inducers. A lightweight emetic for your first aid kit is a small bottle of syrup of ipecac. An adult (about 10 years old or older) gets two tablespoons with eight to sixteen ounces of water. Younger people get one table-spoon with the same amount of water. Do not sit facing them. The vomit tends to come suddenly and forcefully, and may repeat several times. If they haven't vomited in twenty minutes, repeat the dose. After they vomit, activated charcoal can be administered to absorb any remaining poison.

Without ipecac, stimulation of the gag reflex may work to induce vomiting. Lean the patient forward, reach into their mouths with a couple of fingers, and tickle the back of their throat.

DO NOT INDUCE VOMITING IF:

1. They are losing consciousness.
2. They have seizure disorders or heart problems.
3. They have swallowed corrosive acids or bases which can increase damage as they come up.

4. They have swallowed petroleum products which can cause serious pneumonias if even a small amount is breathed into the lungs.

For ingestion of corrosive chemicals or petroleum products, get the patient
to drink a water bottle of water or milk. Diluting the poison can reduce its
effects. It is unlikely you'll be carrying many chemicals in the backcountry. If
someone takes an accidental swallow of gas you brought for the stove, it can
usually be easily managed with dilution. But don't let them smoke for a couple
of hours.

The Barehanded Principles: Poisoning

1. *If they inhaled a poison, remove them from the source. Unless they recover completely and soon, evacuate.*

2. *If they ingested a poison, find out what, when, and how much.*

3. *For ingested poisons, induce vomiting with syrup of ipecac and 8-16 ounces of water unless they swallowed corrosive chemicals or petroleum products, or their level of consciousness is decreasing.*

4. *For ingested corrosive chemicals and petroleum products, dilute the poison with water or milk.*

5. *Evacuate anyone who does not show signs of improvement quickly.*

CHAPTER 27
SEIZURES

Suddenly, there is a great discharge of nervous activity in the cerebral cortex, the "peach pit" part of the brain. There is a episode of involuntary behavior, which may or may not be associated with an altered mental state. Your patient has had a seizure.

It could have been a partial seizure, sometimes called a petit mal seizure. A specific location in the brain is involved, and the patient usually loses contact with reality for a minute or two, and sometimes can be observed to manifest a localized motor movement. The partial seizure may or may not become a generalized, or grand mal, seizure. The generalized seizure can be shocking to watch. Victims usually collapse into rigid, jerky motions of appalling violence. They often stop breathing and turn blue. They often are incontinent, and may bite their tongue.

Although sufferers are commonly referred to as epileptics when the source of the seizures is unknown, the problem may be caused by head injury, heat stroke, diabetes, fever, brain tumor, infection, alcohol or drug withdrawal, and assorted other reasons. Frequent sufferers often experience an aura, a warning signal telling them a seizure is imminent. Your patient is ill, and deserves your compassionate care like all who need help.

A seizure must run its course once it has begun. You can't stop it, but you can protect the victim during the episode. Do not restrain the victim. Move objects away that might cause damage if hit. Cushion under the head with a shirt or parka. They cannot swallow their tongue. Do not try to put anything into the mouth. More epileptics, probably, are harmed by misdirected aid than by the seizure itself.

Stay calm, and comfort the patient once a normal level of consciousness returns. Protect their dignity. They may not be sure what has happened. Don't let the patient drink or move around at first. Most patients will be in a sleepy-recovery phase after the seizure, sometimes called a post-ictal state. Check for injuries that could have occurred.

If they don't regain consciousness immediately after the event, roll them gently onto one side or the other to maintain an adequate airway.

Take some notes on what happened: time, focal areas if you noticed any, length of seizure, triggering events if known.

The greatest danger to a seizure victim is status epilepticus, a persistent seizure or series of seizures with no time for adequate breathing. If this goes on for too long, permanent damage or death may result. There is little or nothing to be done in the backcountry for this person.

A known seizure patient does not need to be evacuated, as long as they are dealing with the situation, and their intended pursuits do not jeopardize their lives. First time seizures, or seizures for unknown reasons, should be evacuated as soon as possible for medical attention.

The Barehanded Principles:
Seizures

1. *Be aware of seizure sufferers, and, if possible, their triggering mechanisms.*
2. *Make sure they are carrying and taking their anti-convulsant medications.*
3. *If a seizure occurs, protect them from harm.*
4. *Do not restrain them.*
5. *Do not put anything in their mouth.*
6. *Protect their dignity.*
7. *Keep them at rest and give them nothing to drink until their level of consciousness returns to normal.*
8. *Maintain an adequate airway for those who do not return immediately to consciousness.*
9. *Check for injuries.*
10. *Evacuate first time seizures, and seizures with unknown sources.*

CHAPTER 28
BLISTERS

Those fluid-filled bubbles are mild second degree burns caused by friction. The friction produces a separation of the tough outer layer of our skin from the sensitive inner layer. Only where skin is hardened is it thick enough for this to happen—heels, soles, palms. Loose skin just wears away with friction leaving an abrasion.

The space between the outer layer of the blister (the roof) and the inner layer (the base) fills with fluid drawn from our circulatory system to protect the damaged area while it heals. Gravity encourages this to happen and causes foot blisters to swell rapidly.

Wet skin blisters much more quickly than dry skin, and warm skin more quickly than cool skin. And what skin is more moist and hot than our feet in heavy boots after a long walk?

On their own, blisters will range from unpleasant to terribly debilitating. But they are not a serious medical problem unless they become infected.

What should you do? Blisters heal faster when the fluid is drained, three to four times faster. Besides, they feel better when the bubble is deflated. Clean around the site thoroughly with soap and water, or alcohol, if either is available. Or wash as best you can with just water. In a flame, sterilize the point of a needle, safety pin, or knife. Puncture the blister a couple of times near its base. Gently massage until the fluid is gone. Leaving the roof intact will let it feel better and mend quicker. If the roof has already been rubbed away when you discover the injury, treat the wound initially as you would any other—clean it and keep it clean to prevent infection.

Now the idea is to reduce the friction on that area as much as possible while staying actively involved in the field. Put a gob of gooey antiseptic on the

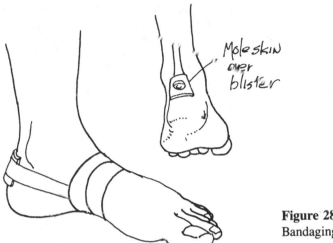

Moleskin over blister

Figure 28–1
Bandaging a blister.

deflated blister. A povidone-iodine ointment works very well. Cover the site with a thick gauze pad, or build a moleskin "donut". Tape the gauze or moleskin securely in place. A liberal application of tincture of benzoin on your skin before the moleskin or tape will greatly increase the stick-to-it-ness of both materials. If you run strips of tape along the sides of the foot, toward the toes, then tape down the ends with strips that run around the instep, your efforts will outlast the abuse further travel puts on the system. More ointment on the outside of the tape will soil your socks but reduce friction even more.

You may never need these directions if you take precautions to prevent blisters from forming. Of critical importance is the fit of your boots. It doesn't matter how expensively your feet are shoed if the fit is poor. Fit your boots with the socks you intend to wear in them. Boots that are the right size and are well broken in go a long way toward preventing blisters.

Keeping your feet cool and dry is important. Take frequent breaks with your boots off. Wear a thin liner sock that wicks moisture away from your feet and into a thicker outer sock. Some folks report success from applications of anti-perspirants to their feet. Most people think it makes their feet sticky which increases friction. Some foot powders help reduce moisture and friction, but they also tend to cake up and require frequent reapplications.

Listen to your feet. When you hear a "hot spot" developing, stop and cover the area with tape or moleskin before the blister has a chance to form. The moleskin will conform to the shape of your feet better if you cut it into strips first instead of laying down a wide piece that inevitably refuses to go flat. Once again, tincture of benzoin applied first will help keep the tape or moleskin from peeling off when your feet start sweating. Without tape or moleskin, benzoi-

can be applied to the skin of feet to prevent blisters. Benzoin hardens the outer layers of skin, and can be applied to hands also to prevent blisters that result from long hours of paddling.

CHAPTER 29
DENTAL EMERGENCIES

He was in pain. He was not in the least bit happy. When I paddled my canoe alongside, his lip had already puffed out as far as his nose, and the broken piece of his tooth lay in his open palm. For Robert, it was a lesson in choosing your paddling partner more carefully. For me, it was a stimulus to learn some basic dentistry for the field.

Backcountry tooth care can be divided into three categories: 1) prevention, 2) oral irritations, and 3) severe tooth pain. Preparing for outdoor toothaches can mean finishing the day's fishing trip, the weekend's hike, or the extended expedition in relative comfort, instead of sacrificing the fun to a throbbing jaw.

PREVENTION: See your dentist regularly, and at least 30 days before an extended trip, giving yourself time to have any discovered problems fixed. Routine oral hygiene includes brushing with a soft nylon bristle toothbrush. Try to eat apples, carrots, or celery regularly. These fibrous fruits and vegetables *after* a meal help scrape teeth clean. And don't forget to floss, cleaning where the brush can't reach.

ORAL IRRITATIONS: Aside from the occasional swat across the mouth with a careless paddle, most people first notice dental pain while eating. The discomfort is often elicited when cold, sweets, or your tongue hits where a filling has fallen out. Gently clean the area, removing any food that may be trapped in the tooth. Dip a cotton pellet in oil of cloves (eugenol) and swab out the vacancy. The pain should be soothed, but to ensure longer lasting results, mix a little zinc oxide powder with a few drops of oil of cloves and stir the stuff until it becomes a paste. Push the paste into the hole. Or carry a tube of Cavit in your first aid kit. A squeeze of the tube sends a bit of pre-mixed paste onto your finger. Roll it into a ball and place it where the filling used to be. Bite it softly into shape. Sugarless gum, chewed to softness, can sometimes be successfull▪

used to plug the hole where a filling fell out. All of these temporary fillings will wash out, requiring you to monitor each regularly. If you're a long way from a dentist, simply replace the temporary when the old one comes out. This same procedure can be followed if you break off a piece of a tooth exposing the underlying structures, and producing pain.

A generalized soreness of the mouth, usually centering in the gums, is often due to poor oral hygiene. This condition should first be treated with salt water rinses (teaspoon of salt in glass of water three to four times a day) and aggressive toothbrushing. If the condition persists, see a dentist for antibiotic therapy.

SEVERE DENTAL PAIN: I believe my teeth are connected directly to my pain center. Aches in other parts of my body I can usually ignore. But screeching toothaches demand complete attention. Infection, exposure of the tooth's pulp, exposure of arteries, veins, or nerves, can create a screamer.

If the tooth is knocked out, pick it up by the top, not the root. Rinse it off, but don't scrub it. Your best chance of saving the fang is by pushing it gently back into the hole from whence it came. Once there, dental wax can hold it in place until a dentist can be found. Without the wax, hold it in place with gentle pressure from your jaw. If it hurts, or refuses to go back in, don't force it. Wrap it in sterile gauze, and hold it in your mouth if possible, but keep it safe for the dental surgeon to attempt a replacement later. A piece of tooth broken off by trauma should likewise be saved. If a blow to the mouth has simply loosened a tooth, dental wax can be used to secure the tooth until it firms up or a dentist is found. (Dental wax softens and disappears in the warmth of the mouth, requiring periodic replacement.)

NEVER put an aspirin on the gum next to an aching tooth. This will cause an acid burn of the gum. It can be severe. Swallow the aspirin, or another pain killer, if you need some relief.

Infection is indicated by a lot of swelling of the gum and cheek around an aching tooth. Gas and pus can be trapped inside the gum, causing extreme pain. If the swelling from infection reaches a major stage, the gum may form an elevated bulge that can turn blue. The patient needs antibiotics, and a dentist. If evacuation is not possible, you might have to consider a gentle stab with a sterile point to release the pressure and drain the infection. This is dangerous and not advisable except in radical circumstances. Likewise, attempting to pull a tooth out of an infected socket is dangerous. Both can cause significant bleeding.

Any bleeding inside the mouth, for any reason, can be given direct pressure. You can do this with a gauze pad you have bitten to hold in place. A moistened tea bag (non-herbal) can be used instead of gauze, and may work better. The tannic acid in tea initiates the formation of clotting. Avoid irritating the wound which can renew the bleeding. Irritants are smoking, extremely hot food, chewing on the "bad" side, and sucking on the wound site.

If a crown breaks off a tooth, clean the crown and coat it with a little oil of cloves. Place it back on the tooth to see if it can be fitted properly. Remove it again, and put a dab of Cavit on the crown. Set it immediately back in place, and bite it gently into position. If it won't fit, pack the tooth with dental wax until you can find a dentist.

A friendly dentist, outdoorsperson or not, should be willing to help you in finding and learning how to use the first aid items specific to dental problems.

Suggested Outdoor Dental Emergency Kit

oil of cloves (eugenol)
cotton pellets
gauze pads
Cavit
dental wax
sugarless gum
aspirin, ibuprofen, or other pain killer
tea bags (non-herbal)

CHAPTER 30
DEHYDRATION AND
WATER DISINFECTION

It looks like you're going to walk right across the sky. The ridge we were following swept up into the blue making you want to just keep climbing. Below us the water of the lake glittered in the sun, spreading out like a sea. Water, water, every where, as the Ancient Mariner had said, and us with no drop to drink. We had forgotten our water bottle. It lay by the tent, back in camp.

A couple of tongues were hanging out, and the water down in the lake smiled up at us, adding weight to our misery. The thirst we were suffering was a sign that our fluid level was already low. The nag of a dry mouth means you should have reached for refreshment long ago. Not especially because you want to, but because you know you need to. Dehydration is probably the major cause of feeling unhealthy in the outdoors.

More of your body is water than not. And that fluid is constantly being lost through urination, respiration, sweating, even crying. The loss is aggravated if you develop diarrhea, vomiting, or bleeding from a nasty wound. You need to maintain your personal water table in order to stay healthy.

What does the water do? It keeps the pressure balanced in and out of your cells so you metabolize nutrients more efficiently and, thus, have more energy. Your kidneys need it to function properly. Otherwise, some of their workload is dumped on your liver, and metabolism slows down even more. Brains are very sensitive to water level changes making dehydration one of the primary sources of headache. Lack of sufficient internal water may lead to poor bowel activity resulting in constipation. With dehydration, your blood volume declines and you're set up for the cold weather problems of hypothermia and frostbite. Water is required to keep the sweating mechanism running smoothly, which allows you to stay cool on the hottest day.

Beyond thirst, fatigue, and headache, your urine output will show that you're dehydrated. It should be ample, and clear or light yellow in color. If you haven't gone for a while, and your urine is dark yellow or orange, you're dehydrated. Advanced signs of water deficiency include lightheadedness and increased heart rate, especially when you first rise from a sitting position. If it goes far enough, your brain will fail to function properly.

How much water do you need? On the average, everyone should drink 8–10 eight-ounce glasses of water each day. That's about two quarts. Water intake should be increased if it is hot and dry, and if you are exercising. And those of us who are overweight need more water. Incidentally, drinking lots of water helps reduce your weight, not increase it.

To be safe, drink four quarts of water every day. If you drink more than you need, it simply means a few more trips to the bushes. Coffee, tea, and non-decaffeinated soft drinks are not satisfactory. They increase fluid loss. Alcohol is especially counter-productive. It draws water out of your cells to dilute the increasing toxicity of your blood. Don't mistakenly think your body will draw all the water it needs from the food you eat. Although we do take in fluid that way, the best source of water is water.

Water Disinfection

Finding that much potable liquid in the backcountry can be a problem. If you don't carry it all in with you, there are three other ways to obtain safe water: pasteurization by heating, halogenation with iodine or chlorine, and filtration.

Boiling is an excellent disinfecting process. If the water is heated until it rolls, anywhere in the continental United States, the heat is enough to kill the protozoas, bacterias, and viruses that harm humans.

Iodine is a safer bet on a long backcountry trip. It is more stable. To be sure water is safe to drink after treating it with iodine, or chlorine, you have to consider variables such as temperature and clarity. Instead of risking a bout with some gastrointestinal illness, buy a bottle of water-disinfecting tablets or crystals, and follow the directions on the label.

All backcountry water filters are not created equal. If you choose filtration as your method of getting safe water, be sure to check on the specific qualifications of your selected filter to do all the things you want it to do.

So don't forget your bottle of water. And if the water is cold, so much the better for it is absorbed into your system faster. Your reward will be a well-hydrated sense of health and accomplishment.

Water Purification
Chemical Purification Methods

Substance	Amount Used	Contact Time
Laundry Bleach 4–6%	2 drops/quart	Let stand 30 minutes

(water should have a slight chlorine odor; if not, repeat dose and let stand an additional 15 minutes)

Halazone Tablets	5 tablets/quart	Let stand 30 minutes

(defective Halazone tablets have an objectionable odor)

Tincture of Iodine 2%	5 drops/qt clear water	30 minutes
10 drops/qt cloudy water		

Potable Aqua	1 tablet/qt clear water	10 minutes
(Globuline-	1 tab/qt cloudy water	20 minutes
Tetraglycine	if very cold	30 minutes
hydroperiodide)		

Crystals of iodine can also be used to prepare a saturated iodine-water solution for use in disinfecting drinking water. Four to eight grams of USP grade iodine crystals can be placed in a 1 ounce glass bottle. Water added to this bottle will dissolve an amount of iodine based upon its temperature. It is this saturated iodine-water solution which is then added to the quart of water. The amount added to produce a final concentration of 4 ppm will vary according to temperature as indicated in the chart:

Temperature	Volume	Capfuls*
37 °F (3 °C)	20.0cc	8
68 °F (20 °C)	13.0cc	5+
77 °F (25 °C)	12.5cc	5
104 °F (40 °C)	10.0cc	4

*Assuming $2^1/_2$cc capacity for a standard 1 ounce glass bottle cap.

This water should be stored for 15 minutes before drinking. If the water is turbid, or otherwise contaminated, the amounts of saturated iodine solution indicated above should be doubled and the resultant water stored 20 minutes before using. This product is now commercially available as Polar Pure through many outdoor stores and catalog houses.

Filter systems exist, but water should be pre-treated before using to prevent filter contamination. An exception is the ceramic filter, the Katadyn Pocket

Filter system, which while it will not become contaminated will become plugged and require occasional scraping with a special brush.

Bringing water to a boil will effectively kill germs and make water safe to drink. One reads variously to boil water 5, 10, even 20 minutes. But simply bringing the water temperature to 150 °F (65.5 °C) is adequate to kill all water borne germs. At high altitude the boiling point of water is reduced. For example, at 25,000 feet the boiling point of water would be about 185 °F (85 °C), still quite adequate to prepare safe drinking water.

DESERT SOLAR STILL

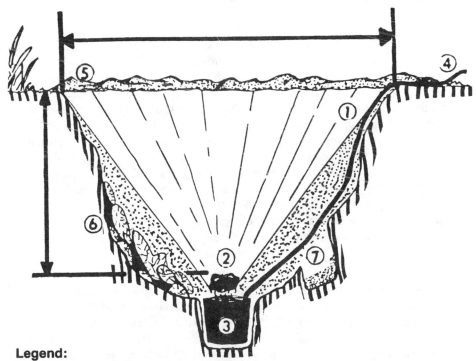

Legend:
1. Sheet of wettable plastic, 6 foot diameter.
2. Smooth, fist sized rock for forming cone of plastic.
3. Pail, jar, can, or cone of soil, plastic or canvas to catch water.
4. Drinking tube, 1/4 inch plastic, about 5 feet long.
   (Desirable but not necessary.)
5. Soil to weight plastic sheet and seal space. A good closure is important.
6. Line hole with broken cacti or other succulents.
7. If non-potable water is available, dig a soaking trough around inside of hole. Carefully fill the trough to prevent impure water from running down and contaminating the water-catching container.

CHAPTER 31
GASTROINTESTINAL DISTRESS

Trips to the wild outdoors with the accompanying change of diet, less than sterile cooking procedures, water from more directly natural sources, even the emotional stress of a new environment, can cause a "stomachache". It is typically a trivial problem, but it can ruin a wilderness experience, for the sufferer and those others who must also endure the sufferer's suffering. The problem can be diarrhea, constipation, nausea, gas, or combinations thereof.

The gastrointestinal tract starts at the mouth and drops down the esophagus. The esophagus lies flat against the back of the windpipe until a swallow and a series of muscular contractions pushes something down it. Passing through the diaphragm, the something enters the stomach. From there the tract wanders through the small intestine until it joins the large intestine in the lower right hand corner of the abdomen. The journey continues upward, then across the upper abdomen, then down to the exit. When the normal function of the tract is disturbed, you are dealing with gastrointestinal distress.

Diarrhea

Diarrhea, the word, comes from the Greek for "a flowing through". Diarrhea, the distress, can come from viruses, bacteria (as in food poisoning), protozoa (like Giardia), and just being very anxious. It can be mild, moderate, or severe depending on the frequency of the rush to the bushes, the pain of cramping, the vileness of gas (judge for yourself), and the wateriness of the bowel movement. The problem can last from six hours to three weeks.

Initial treatment for all diarrhea is essentially the same. Discover what is causing the problem and quit swallowing it, and replace the fluids that are being lost. For fluid replacement clear liquids are the best choice: water, broths, herbal teas, fruit juices you can see through. The diarrhea should go away in about a day.

For a more persistent problem, start replacing the electrolytes that are being lost with the diarrhea. Commercially prepared powders can be carried in your first aid kit, or you can create a field remedy by adding one pinch of salt and one-half to one teaspoon of sugar (and an optional one-half teaspoon of baking soda) to a quart of water. Three to four quarts of this solution every day should be enough.

Non-prescription anti-diarrhea tablets can be carried in your first aid kit, and used with relative safety (read the label). More powerful drugs, the ones that inhibit bowel activity, also trap whatever is causing the diarrhea inside the body. Our body wants to flush out the trouble makers. On extended trips, stronger medications might be advisable, but get advise from your doctor.

Treatment can be augmented by controlling what the sufferer eats. If the diarrhea is persistent, stick to liquids. As the problem subsides, start eating bland foods such as toast, crackers, pasta, rice, potatoes, and avoid spices, alcohol, coffee, fruits, hard cheeses and other fat-laden foods. As the future brightens, add meats and vegetables, but continue to go easy on the irritating foods.

Evacuation is seldom required, but should be undertaken if the patient persistently vomits, develops a fever, complains of a localizing burning pain, or produces dark or black blood in the stool or vomit.

Help prevent diarrhea by maintaining a backcountry diet high in fiber and low in fat. Drink plenty of water, and take precautions to ensure it is disinfected by boiling, filtering, or iodizing. Wash your hands before preparing food, and clean up the kitchen gear after meals.

Constipation

Constipation is a plug in the system usually created by either a fluid level too low to lubricate the tract, a fiber level too low to keep things rolling along, or a poor attitude concerning squatting over a cathole. Constipation can be encouraged by poor exercise habits.

Treatment, as with diarrhea, should start with forcing fluids. Encourage the sufferer to eat lots of whole grains, fruits (dried is OK), and vegetables. Peanut butter, cheese, and high-fat foods should be avoided. If one is prone to the problem, add a stool softener to your first aid kit. Refrain from using the stronger medications for constipation. They can result in explosive deliveries and heavy fluid loss.

Someone who hasn't had a bowel movement in five days could be developing serious problems from the toxins building up their intestinal tract. They should be considered for an evacuation. When evacuation is not an immediate option, it might be necessary to go in with an index finger, break up the impaction, and pull it out. Disgusting as it may sound, it might prove lifesaving.

Prevention of constipation is essentially the same as with diarrhea. Drink plenty of water, eat healthy. For those who have trouble going without a porcelain toilet, try picking a secluded spot with a scenic view and a minimum of tickling grasses . . . and practice.

Nausea

It can come from something you ate, the rocking motion of the boat, or a serious underlying illness. Typically it is just the body's way of dealing with something that is upsetting the normal balance. Nausea would deserve evacuation if it produced persistent vomiting, especially if there is dark "coffee grounds" blood in the vomitus. Reasons for concern also include localized pain and a fever in an overly anxious patient.

Gas

Passing gas rectally (flatus) is usually a relief and often a pleasant experience for the passer. If it becomes a problem, the distress will likely be social instead of medical. Heavy collections of gas can become painful, especially at higher altitudes. An easing of the pain is possible with an antacid containing the drug simethicone, available over the counter.

CHAPTER 32
THE FIVE COMMANDMENTS OF
FIRST AID KITS

NUMBER ONE: Thou shalt find it impossible to put together the perfect first aid kit.

Go ahead and try, but eventually, if you spend enough time in the backcountry, you will one day wish for something that is not there. It is possible to create a kit to meet your every need—almost! But don't ever try to convince someone else that your choice of first aid items is better than theirs. Accept the fact that these kits are very personal. You may get by for years on a small piece of moleskin because your feet are tough. Your partner may need a mile of the stuff for an overnight hike. Not following this principle, here is a list of items for the "almost perfect" first aid kit.

Start with a smallish Zip-loc bag because 1) they're cheap, and 2) they're lightweight, and 3) they're see-through so you don't have to dump everything out on the ground to find what you need. What you might be dumping in the dirt should include:

. . . About a half-dozen band-aids. The ones that are somewhat resistant to water last longer, and the ones about 1 x 3 inches work in most situations. Remember they go on after a wound has been thoroughly cleaned to protect it and keep the dirt out.

. . . A couple of sterile gauze pads, around 4 x 4 inches. They'll cover larger ouchies, and can be cut down for smaller wounds, and doubled up for bigger ones. They can be used to scrub out dirtier injuries, or molded into a covering for an irritated eye.

. . . A roll of athletic tape, 1 inch x 10 yards. It holds down the gauze, prevents blisters when applied to sensitive spots at the start of a trip, and repairs injured equipment for short periods of time. Athletic tape shapes itself more easily to the strange designs of human extremities, and can be used to supportively wrap ankles if you know how.

. . . A small bottle of tincture of benzoin. When the benzoin is rubbed on skin before tape is applied, the tape sticks better.

. . . A couple of butterfly band-aids or steri-strips. These are for pulling together the sides of a clean wound that gapes open, until a doctor can be found.

. . . An individually wrapped sanitary napkin. This lightweight, inexpensive item makes a wonderful compress for badly bleeding injuries.

. . . A tube of povidone-iodine ointment. It can be used directly from the tube to disinfect wounds, or dissolved in water to make a solution for washing or soaking injuries. A dab of the jelly-like substance dissolved in a liter of water creates a disinfected drink if other means of cleaning up water are not available. It will work for short periods of time as a lubricant on abraded areas of a body. It also temporarily turns skin orange.

. . . moleskin, a piece 4 x 4 inches or so. It works great to prevent blisters if applied before the damage is done, and can be cut into "donuts" to treat blisters so a trip can continue in more comfort after a bubble has developed.

. . . A few tablets of a painkiller. This medication can bring a bit of relief after you have grown a headache, a muscle or joint ache, a fever, or just about anything that causes painful discomfort.

. . . A six-inch wide elastic wrap. Ace makes the most popular brand. The bandage can be used to compress strains and sprains for a little added comfort, or used to hold a possible broken bone to a splint, or used as a constricting band in the treatment of poisonous snakebite, or used to hold the compress on a bad bleed, or used in any other creative way you can think of.

. . . A couple of safety pins. They can secure the elastic wrap, be sterilized and puncture a blister to drain it, repair rips in clothing, or whatever.

. . . A few mild antihistamine tablets. Benadryl is probably the best for most people. Their sedative effect helps relieve the itch of allergies and insect bites, helps you get to sleep (so don't take one and continue a high-risk outdoor activity), and helps ease the symptoms of a cold (but antihistamines do not cure a runny nose, and possibly extend the cold's life by causing your body to forget to fight off the infection).

. . . A couple of tablets of Pepto-Bismol will come in handy if something upsets your stomach.

. . . A small set of scissors and tweezers are things you'll find yourself using on a daily basis in the backcountry. They can be a part of your pocketknife, which is the friendliest way to keep them ready for use.

Throw in other items depending on the time of year and the part of the country you're traveling through. Things like a dab of meat tenderizer to rub on serious insect bites, sunscreen, alcohol to soften attached ticks before removal, lip balm, more potent medications for specific problems, and the phone numbers of the closest emergency aid in case something really bad happens and you have to hurry out for help.

You have most likely already thought of things that should have been left out or included. Fine! Put them all in a bag, and carry it whenever you travel outdoors. A first aid kit is only useful if it's with you.

NUMBER TWO: Thou shalt choose things for your first aid kit that are versatile rather than specific. You do not need to carry on your back a variety of different sizes of band-aids, several widths of tape, three brands of painkillers (in their original bottles), and a wide range of thicknesses of gauze. Pack a few of the most commonly used shapes and sizes of the most commonly used items, and make do if a odd-shaped boo-boo occurs.

NUMBER THREE: Thou shalt not carry anything in your first aid kit that you are not familiar with.

What's the point of packing along something you don't know how to use? Why carry a suture kit or prescription drugs unless you fully understand their uses? Besides, it could be dangerous for the person who needs first aid if you try to sew up a gaping wound, or give them some medications they can't tolerate.

NUMBER FOUR: Thou shalt re-pack your first aid kit at least seasonally.

For one thing, there are expiration dates on many of those containers of medicinal supplies. And for another thing, moisture or heat or cold can creep in and destroy the efficacy of some of your items, and you'll never know it until you reach for them. Finally, lazy kit-checkers find they're carrying insect repellent on a winter trip where it is useless. Or rubbing alcohol on an ski excursion where it can be dangerous. What you include in your kit may also change when you explore a new geographic location.

NUMBER FIVE: Thou shalt not forget that the first aid kit that saves lives is not made of items stuffed in a Zip-loc bag but skills carried in the human brain.

Kits are for the little trivial injuries that would probably be OK whether you interfere or not. Your ministrations can ease pain and speed healing, but it is knowledge and the ability to use that knowledge that makes the difference between life and death in a critical situation. Learn what to do for the seriously hurt or sick person, and carry that information with you at all times.

INDEX

157